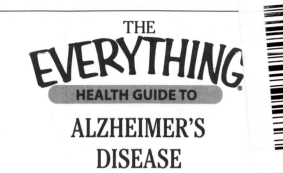

THE
EVERYTHING®
HEALTH GUIDE TO
ALZHEIMER'S DISEASE

Dear Reader,

Dementia is a devastating illness. No one who watches a loved one go through it should have to scramble to find resources, advice, or support. But many spouses, children, and friends of people with Alzheimer's spend valuable time doing just that.

Some take on roles that range from health care proxy to errand runner. Others serve as interpreters, legal advocates, or food testers. Professional reporters and avid researchers, like me, turn into hunter-gatherers, seeking health care or long-term housing information, digging for legal expertise, or tracking down blood test results.

Despite all our efforts, our loved ones gradually, steadily slip away. The tremendous task of making sure someone with Alzheimer's is safe, comfortable, and reasonably content each day is an astonishingly difficult enterprise. But some part of it should be easier than it is. I've started with information gathering. It's all here, in one place.

Maureen Dezell

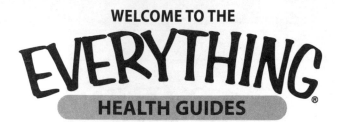

WELCOME TO THE
EVERYTHING®
HEALTH GUIDES

Everything® Health Guides are a part of the bestselling Everything® series and cover important health topics like anxiety, postpartum care, and thyroid disease. Packed with the most recent, up-to-date data, Everything® Health Guides help you get the right diagnosis, choose the best doctor, and find the treatment options that work for you. With this one comprehensive resource, you and your family members have all the information you need right at your fingertips.

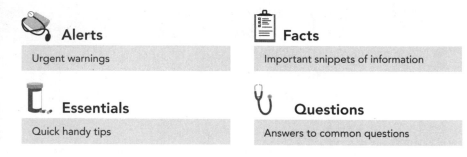

Alerts
Urgent warnings

Facts
Important snippets of information

Essentials
Quick handy tips

Questions
Answers to common questions

When you're done reading, you can finally say you know **EVERYTHING®**!

PUBLISHER Karen Cooper

DIRECTOR OF ACQUISITIONS AND INNOVATION Paula Munier

MANAGING EDITOR, EVERYTHING® SERIES Lisa Laing

COPY CHIEF Casey Ebert

ACQUISITIONS EDITOR Katrina Schroeder

ASSOCIATE DEVELOPMENT EDITOR Elizabeth Kassab

EDITORIAL ASSISTANT Hillary Thompson

EVERYTHING® SERIES COVER DESIGNER Erin Alexander

LAYOUT DESIGNERS Colleen Cunningham, Elisabeth Lariviere, Ashley Vierra, Denise Wallace

Visit the entire Everything® series at *www.everything.com*

THE
EVERYTHING®

HEALTH GUIDE TO

ALZHEIMER'S DISEASE

A reassuring, informative guide
for families and caregivers

Maureen Dezell with Carrie Hill, PhD

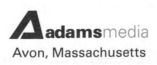

Avon, Massachusetts

In memory of Eileen Sullivan Dezell

An Everything® Series Book.
Everything® and everything.com® are registered trademarks of F+W Media, Inc.

Published by Adams Media, a division of F+W Media, Inc.
57 Littlefield Street, Avon, MA 02322 U.S.A.
www.adamsmedia.com

ISBN 10: 1-60550-124-7
ISBN 13: 978-1-60550-124-6

Printed in the United States of America.

J I H G F E D C B A

Library of Congress Cataloging-in-Publication Data
is available from the publisher.

Some of the anecdotes and examples in this book appear in composite, fictional-ized vignettes that are based on experiences of people living with Alzheimer's. In these accounts, individual speakers are quoted by first name only.

Acknowledgments

Thank you once again to John for seeing me through. Special thanks to Beth McGowan, Tom Dezell, and Father Ray Sullivan for helping Mom through. Love and thanks to Christopher, too.

Contents

Introduction

Every seventy-one seconds, someone in the United States develops Alzheimer's disease (AD). In 2050, Alzheimer's will strike every thirty-three seconds if no cure is found for the progressive, fatal brain disease. Like most statistics about Alzheimer's, these are staggering—more so because recent surveys show that while half of Americans say they have been touched by someone with Alzheimer's, a majority underestimate the prevalence and impact of this insidious disease.

Nearly one-third of American adults, for example, think there are approximately 1 million Alzheimer's sufferers in the United States, according to a 2009 Harris Interactive Census conducted for HBO's *The Alzheimer's Project*. In fact, at least 5 million Americans are afflicted. The Harris census and a 2007 Alzheimer's Association survey showed that few people know that AD is a leading cause of death in the United States, that it is difficult to diagnose, or that it is the third most expensive disease to treat after heart disease and cancer.

American adults fear Alzheimer's more than heart disease, stroke, or diabetes, according to a 2006 MetLife Foundation survey.

That may explain why a substantial majority (65 percent) acknowledge that they joke about Alzheimer's, but only half of those who responded to the Alzheimer's Association survey knew that people lose control of their bodies and die from AD. Approximately one in three Americans worries about getting Alzheimer's, according to the Harris survey. The truth is, many Americans will develop Alzheimer's or care for someone who has it during their lifetimes. Ours is an aging society, and Alzheimer's is primarily a disease affecting older people.

An estimated 5 million people sixty-five and older suffer now from Alzheimer's, and 10 million baby boomers are poised to get it, according to federal health statistics. By 2030, the number of afflicted people over sixty-five is expected to rise to 7.7 million—more than a 50 percent increase from today. The Alzheimer's Association estimates that some 70 percent of Alzheimer's patients live with their families, and 10 million American adults provide "free" at-home AD care.

Alzheimer's will soon prove impossible to ignore. In 1995 an estimated 377,000 new cases of Alzheimer's were diagnosed each year. By 2000, that number had risen to 411,000 cases. An estimated 500,000 are diagnosed annually today, and that number could double to close to 1 million cases per year by 2050, according to the Centers for Disease Control and Prevention (CDC). Alzheimer's disease threatens to engulf the Medicare system by 2030, when AD alone will cost the federal health insurer $400 billion—nearly as much as the entire current Medicare budget, according to the Alzheimer's Association.

There is no cure for Alzheimer's on the horizon, nor is there a magic bullet to treat it, though several interesting theories on detecting and managing the disease are under investigation. But research and development of new treatments and techniques also demand investment of time and human capital.

Scientific understanding of AD is progressing, and researchers maintain they are making significant strides toward diagnosing, treating, and preventing the disease.

But as the number of AD diagnoses has risen, funding for Alzheimer's research and development has been flat. Only public awareness and advocacy will change that. Presented with the facts about Alzheimer's, 72 percent of survey participants said they would be willing to help raise funds for an Alzheimer's cure.

CHAPTER 1

The Alzheimer's Disease Dilemma

More than 5 million people in the United States have Alzheimer's disease (AD), a degenerative, incurable brain disease that systematically robs the mind of its ability to think, plan, remember, and express basic thoughts and needs. As of 2010, a half million new cases of AD are diagnosed each year. The number of people living with Alzheimer's will grow exponentially as Americans live longer and healthier lives. This poses phenomenal challenges to individuals, their families, the public health system, and our society as a whole.

Alzheimer's Disease: A Brief History

Every seventy-one seconds, someone in America develops Alzheimer's disease. By mid-century, someone will develop Alzheimer's every thirty-three seconds. But what exactly is the disease?

Dr. Alois Alzheimer

Alzheimer's disease is the most common cause of dementia—a clinical disorder characterized by a loss of memory and other cognitive abilities. It is named for Dr. Alois Alzheimer, the early-twentieth-century German physician who reported brain abnormalities in a patient who suffered from a strange, severe dementia.

In 1901, a fifty-one-year-old woman known as Mrs. Auguste D. entered a Frankfurt asylum, where she was put under Dr. Alzheimer's care. The patient's memory loss was debilitating. She had difficulty speaking and understanding what was said to her. She grew suspicious, then paranoid, convinced her husband was unfaithful. Her condition deteriorated. "I have lost myself," Mrs. D. told her doctor. Five years after she entered the hospital, she was bedridden and helpless. She died from pneumonia and infections from bedsores.

An autopsy on Mrs. D's brain revealed damage unlike any Alzheimer had seen. At a scientific meeting in 1906, he described the dramatic shrinkage of the brain, particularly the cortex, the gray matter involved in memory, thinking, judgment, and speech. He also described abnormal "clumps," now known as *amyloid plaques*, and knots, called *neurofibrillary tangles*, that are considered telltale indicators of Alzheimer's disease.

Fact

Alzheimer's accounts for 70 percent of all dementia cases among Americans age seventy-one and older. Vascular dementia accounts for 17 percent of dementia cases, and diseases such as Parkinson's, Lewy body dementia, and frontotemporal dementia make up the remaining 13 percent.

No one is sure whether the buildup of plaques and tangles in the brain is a cause or effect of Alzheimer's disease. What is certain is that plaques and tangles destroy brain cells and disrupt communication pathways essential to normal brain activity.

The Mid-Twentieth Century

"Senile dementia" was long considered a normal part of aging and was treated as such. It was not until the 1950s that scientists began to study the biological structure of the plaques and tangles

Alzheimer had noticed. In the 1960s, researchers connected plaque in the brain to dementia and recognized Alzheimer's as a distinct disease, although it was not until the 1980s that diagnostic criteria were outlined in the American Psychiatric Association's *Diagnostic and Statistical Manual of Mental Disorders*. Further research in the 1970s revealed that chemicals in the brains of patients with Alzheimer's undergo changes; these findings led to additional breakthroughs in understanding the disease. In the 1990s, genetic mutations were linked to Alzheimer's.

Recent Developments

In 1993, Cognex, the first drug to treat cognitive symptoms of Alzheimer's, was approved by the FDA. A new generation of drugs—rivastigmine (Exelon), galantamine (Razadyne), donepezil (Aricept), and memantine (Namenda)—earned FDA approval to treat symptoms of Alzheimer's between 1998 and 2006. Researchers are trying to develop new drugs and a vaccine for Alzheimer's.

Efforts to definitively diagnose the disease are also progressing. In 2004 and 2005, researchers published the results of groundbreaking studies that allowed doctors to see plaques in the brains of living patients using positron emission tomography scans (PET scans). Increasingly sophisticated neuroimaging techniques, breakthroughs in ongoing research into the genetics of Alzheimer's, and other advances continue to improve doctors' ability to identify people at high risk for AD.

Who Is at Risk for AD?

One in six women and one in ten men who live to be at least fifty-five will develop Alzheimer's disease in their remaining lifetimes. The risk of developing Alzheimer's is higher for women than for men because women typically live longer. One in eight Americans age sixty-five or older and nearly half of those over eighty-five had Alzheimer's in 2008, the year AD surpassed diabetes as the sixth leading cause of death in the United States, according to the Centers for Disease Control and Prevention (CDC).

 Alert

Thanks to advances in medical care and treatment, death rates from 2000 to 2005 declined for most major diseases, including heart disease (-8.6 percent), breast cancer (-8 percent), prostate cancer (-4.9 percent), and stroke (-14.4 percent), according to the CDC. Alzheimer's disease death rates increased 45 percent during the same time period.

By 2000, an estimated 411,000 new cases of Alzheimer's disease were diagnosed each year. That number has risen to nearly half a million annually and could double to as many as 1 million cases a year by 2050, according to the CDC.

An estimated 10 million baby boomers are expected to develop Alzheimer's during the next thirty years. By 2030, nearly one out of five Americans will be over sixty-five. In that year, the number of people age sixty-five and over with Alzheimer's disease is expected to reach 7.7 million, an increase of more than 50 percent over the number of Alzheimer's patients today.

Symptoms of Alzheimer's

AD strikes first in brain memory centers, and its initial and most recognized symptoms usually involve short-term memory loss, such as forgetfulness and difficulty learning new information. But disorientation and language problems are common symptoms that are often overlooked.

Signs to Look For

Alzheimer's goes beyond memory. It affects language, learning, and judgment, notes Martin J. Gorbien, MD, director of geriatric medicine at Rush University Medical Center. Gorbien encourages people who are concerned about memory loss to pay attention to symptoms that are frequently mistaken for other conditions, including the following:

- Periods of forgetfulness that persist and get worse over time. A tendency to misplace things, often in peculiar places. Difficulty recalling names of friends, family, and everyday objects. Language and communication problems. Trouble finding the right words to express thoughts. Difficulty following directions or even conversations.
- Problems with abstract thinking, particularly calculation. Trouble balancing the checkbook and dealing with numbers.
- Disorientation about time, dates, and familiar surroundings. Inability to remember appointments or whether and when to take medicine.
- Impaired judgment. Knowing what to do if food on the stove is burning or the car is "missing" becomes increasingly difficult, and eventually impossible. Familiar activities and tasks, such as cooking, become harder to handle.
- Difficulty doing things that require planning and making decisions (e.g., planning a meal or choosing a health care plan).
- Personality changes. Mood swings. Depression. Suspicious behavior. Stubbornness and withdrawal.

How Long Does Alzheimer's Last?

Alzheimer's begins to develop years before its symptoms appear and can last anywhere from two to twenty years after that. People with Alzheimer's live for an average of eight years after diagnosis. Most experts divide the progress of AD into three general stages—mild (or early-stage), moderate (or mid-stage), and severe (or late-stage) AD.

In early-stage Alzheimer's, many people can live independently. But as the disease progresses, memory loss, confusion, and disorientation become increasingly problematic. Mid-stage patients need more assistance and grow dependent on others for help performing daily activities and meeting basic needs such as bathing, dressing, using the bathroom, and eating.

As the end of life approaches, most Alzheimer's patients lose all ability to communicate. They are unaware of their surroundings and unable to recognize loved ones. People with Alzheimer's gradually lose their ability to coordinate basic motor skills such as walking, controlling their bladders, and even swallowing. They are prone to infection and susceptible to diseases such as pneumonia, which can be caused by bacteria, infection, or inhaling food or fluid (because a patient has difficulty swallowing). People with late-stage Alzheimer's are prone to falls and fractures from which they seldom recover, because they have lost the capacity to follow directions and the motivation to get better. Bed-bound, they require round-the-clock care. Most people die with Alzheimer's, not from it. The most common causes of death are usually listed as pneumonia or infection.

What Causes Alzheimer's?

Scientists don't know yet what causes Alzheimer's disease. Most agree it is probably triggered by a combination of age, genetics, environment, and lifestyle factors.

Question

What is early-onset Alzheimer's?
Early-onset Alzheimer's disease is a rare form of AD that strikes people between the ages of thirty and sixty-five. It accounts for approximately 10 percent of all cases in the United States, according to the Alzheimer's Association. Approximately half of early-onset cases run in families and are linked to three rare genes that cause Alzheimer's.

Though Alzheimer's is not an inevitable or normal part of aging, there is no question that growing older greatly increases the risk of developing the disease. At age sixty-five, you have at least a one in ten chance of developing Alzheimer's. The risk doubles every five years after that. At age eighty-five, the risk for AD is one in two.

Scientists are beginning to uncover clues to genetic influences in early- and late-onset Alzheimer's. Many suspect that diet, fitness levels, and lifestyle factors that put you at risk for diabetes and heart disease may also influence whether you get AD.

DIAGNOSIS

"I really try not to hold on to negative feelings. But I am still angry at how many hoops I had to go through to get a diagnosis," says Suzanna, who was diagnosed with early-onset Alzheimer's in 2007, when she was fifty-three.

A retired health care executive, she first consulted her internist about "weird memory and language problems" right around her fiftieth birthday. "I then spent three years going from doctor to doctor, specialist to specialist, scary test to scary test," she says.

"In some places, it's tough to find specialists. In Boston, where I live, you have medical specialists galore. Everyone I saw was a top expert in some part of the brain or body or nervous system. But none of them saw all of me or all my symptoms."

Suzanna was treated at different points with anti-anxiety drugs, anti-depressants, and hormone therapy. A neurologist who suspected Lyme disease prescribed a course of antibiotics. She also underwent batteries of tests, which were time-consuming, distressing—and ultimately inconclusive.

Meanwhile, her symptoms got worse. "I was having trouble remembering things and saying things. There was one week when my secretary whispered to me something like, 'You told me that twice. Are you okay?' A few days later, I was talking to my son on the phone, trying to remind him to lock the door. I couldn't remember the word for door! I think I said something like 'secure the entryway.'"

At that point, Suzanna called her neurologist and demanded an emergency appointment. "I said, 'Okay, you know my symptoms. They don't fit depression or menopause or Lyme disease. What do they fit?'

"Unfortunately, the answer was Alzheimer's," Suzanne says. "But knowing it let me get on with life!"

How Is Alzheimer's Diagnosed and Treated?

Alzheimer's can only be confirmed with 100 percent certainty during an autopsy. But physicians who are familiar with the disease can usually diagnose it with 90 percent accuracy through a process of elimination. The process usually includes a complete medical history, a physical examination, a mental status test, and blood work. Some physicians also order neuropsychological testing and brain imaging scans to confirm or rule out suspected AD.

The U.S. Food and Drug Administration (FDA) has approved four drugs that help slow cognitive decline associated with Alzheimer's. Overall, the medications are considered moderately effective in some patients for a limited time—usually a year or less. Doctors sometimes prescribe other drugs to improve symptoms that often accompany Alzheimer's, including sleeplessness, wandering, anxiety, agitation, and depression.

The Costs of Alzheimer's

The annual national direct and indirect costs of caring for people with Alzheimer's is at least $100 billion, according to the National

Institute on Aging. That number is only expected to rise as the number of Alzheimer's patients increases.

Staggering Statistics

People with Alzheimer's and other dementias are hospitalized three times as often as other older people, in part because many also suffer other serious medical conditions, such as diabetes and congestive heart failure. Medicare, the federal health insurance program for people age sixty-five and older, spends more than three times as much for individuals with Alzheimer's and other dementias as it does for the average Medicare beneficiary, according to the U.S. Department of Health and Human Services.

In 2005, Medicare spent $91 billion on Alzheimer's and dementia care and treatment. By 2010, Alzheimer's care will cost Medicare approximately $160 billion annually, according to projections. By 2015, the tab will be $189 billion.

 Alert

In 2007, nearly 10 million Americans age eighteen and over provided 8.4 billion hours of unpaid care worth $89 billion to people with Alzheimer's disease, according to the Alzheimer's Association. The organization calculated the market value rate of unpaid care based on an hourly wage of $10.58 per hour, which is the average of the minimum wage ($5.85 per hour) and the average wage of a home health care aide in July 2007 ($15.32 per hour).

By 2030, Medicare spending on Alzheimer's patients alone may cost nearly $400 billion—roughly equivalent to today's entire Medicare budget, according to the Alzheimer's Association. Health experts warn that paying for AD could bankrupt the federal health budget.

Medicare spending was projected to be 3.3 percent of the gross domestic product (GDP) in 2009. It is expected to grow to 7.3 percent of GDP by 2035.

Covering the Costs

Federal government spending on Alzheimer's research and development failed to keep pace with the escalation of the disease for much of the past decade. Between 1998 and 2003, Congress doubled total funding for the National Institutes of Health (NIH), providing a steady increase in Alzheimer research funding. But NIH appropriations for the subsequent five years (fiscal years 2004 through 2009) was stagnant, and the NIH research appropriations budget, adjusted for inflation, actually dipped by approximately 13 percent, according to the American Association for the Advancement of Science.

As a result, good science went unfunded, young scientists were discouraged from pursuing dementia research, and life-saving treatments were delayed, according to the Alzheimer's Association.

What's more, there were notable discrepancies in spending on individual diseases. In 2008, the federal government allocated $644 million, or $124 per American patient, to Alzheimer's disease. By comparison, funding for HIV/AIDS that year was $2.9 billion, or $3,052 per patient.

The American Recovery and Reinvestment Act, which Congress enacted in 2009, provided $8.7 billion overall for NIH research and research-related activities, including what Congress called "significant expansion in cutting-edge research to study diseases such as Alzheimer's, Parkinson's, cancer, and heart disease."

Federal funding for AD research and development was expected to increase under the Obama administration, and federal agencies were reviewing the policies for spending on individual diseases.

SHARING INFORMATION AND ADVICE

When her dad developed memory problems that were "maybe Alzheimer's, maybe a stroke, maybe something else," Mona Johnson started digging for information and explanations of memory loss. Two aunts had had dementia, and she wanted to know more—much more—about the disease.

A telecom industry executive and writer, Mona struggled to "piece together enough information to help Mom talk with the doctors." Mona and her sister searched the Internet. Their brother, a professor of library science, sent references.

Before he died in late 2005, Mona's father urged her to continue her research and to "write this stuff." He told her she was "smart enough to talk with the doctors and scientists and write about it so people can understand."

Fortunately, Johnson took her dad's advice. Today, she writes "The Tangled Neuron: A Layperson Reports on Memory Loss, Alzheimer's & Dementia" (*www.tangledneuron.info*), an accessible, evidence-based report on medical, scientific, and government information about memory loss and dementia.

Johnson's website is informed, balanced, and up-to date. She reports good news and breakthroughs as they occur. She also writes candidly and clearly about failed drug trials and disappointing research developments that have dampened scientific optimism about Alzheimer's in the past few years.

"When my father started to have problems with his memory, my understanding of Alzheimer's was that it was a single and identifiable disease, and that we were close to finding a cure," Johnson told her readers in early 2009. That was the essence of scientific thinking in 2005, when the National Institute on Aging expected success in what it called a "vigorous assault" in the "fight against AD." Unfortunately, what is now clear to experts, Johnson, and her readers is that Alzheimer's has no single cause but develops from multiple factors over many years.

CHAPTER 2

What Is Alzheimer's Disease?

Alzheimer's disease is the most common form of dementia, a general term used to describe the loss of memory and other intellectual abilities severe enough to interfere with day-to-day life. Alzheimer's is not a normal part of aging. It is progressive and incurable, a debilitating condition that slowly destroys memory, intellect, and personality. Eventually, it renders its sufferers helpless. Scientists aren't sure what causes Alzheimer's, but they do know its symptoms, how they develop, and the ways they affect the body and brain.

What We Know about What Goes Wrong

Alzheimer's wreaks havoc by destroying nerve cells, causing widespread neuron death throughout the brain. As neurons die, damaged areas of the brain begin to atrophy, or shrink. Widespread nerve cell death is what destroys memory, personality, and brain and body function.

As explained in Chapter 1, Dr. Alois Alzheimer, the German neurologist for whom the disease is named, identified two brain abnormalities—now called *plaques* and *tangles*—that distinguish Alzheimer's from other dementias. Amyloid plaques are made up of deposits of beta-amyloid protein mixed with other proteins and bits and pieces of nerve cells. Plaques build up between nerve cells, where they are believed to block normal cell communication. Neurofibrillary tangles, which are twisted threads of a protein called *tau*, develop inside neurons, preventing normal nerve cell function and causing cells to die.

Fact

Most people develop some plaques and tangles as they grow older. People with AD build up more than most, and theirs tend to develop in a predictable pattern, beginning in areas of the brain critical to learning and memory before spreading to other regions.

Low levels of certain brain chemicals, especially acetylcholine, a neurotransmitter important in memory, are also characteristics of Alzheimer's disease.

The Healthy Brain

Changes in the brains of people with Alzheimer's begin decades before the disease is diagnosed. Nerve destruction starts in the hippocampus and other areas essential to memory, learning, and spatial orientation. It then takes a predictable, relentless path through the brain. However, it progresses at very different rates in different individuals.

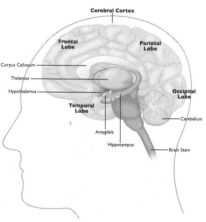

Brain Basics

Most illustrations of the normal, three-pound brain show its distinct parts:

- The brain stem is the smallest and most primitive structure. The brain stem connects the brain and spinal cord, the two parts of the central nervous system. It also regulates essential body functions we usually don't think about, such as heart rate, breathing, digestion, blood pressure, and sweating.
- The cerebellum controls balance and coordination. This is the part of the brain that allows us to swim, hit a tennis ball, sit up straight, and walk without thinking.
- The cerebrum is the largest, most evolved part of the brain. Divided into two hemispheres, the cerebrum fills approximately 80 percent of the human skull. The left hemisphere controls the right side of your body. The right hemisphere rules the left. Though the hemispheres seem to mirror one another, scientists think language ability is largely located in the left hemisphere, and abstract thought and reasoning in the right. The hemispheres communicate with one another through the corpus callosum, a bundle of nerve fibers.
- The cortex is a wrinkled-looking layer of gray matter less than ¼-inch thick that surrounds the cerebral hemispheres. It is the brain's center of intellect, language, and consciousness. The cerebral cortex is where you see and interpret the world. It's where you think, reason, and imagine. The cerebral cortex is what makes us human.

About Those Lobes

Experts have compared the brain to an ecosystem of living organisms. Continually engaged in multiple relationships with one another, each and all are vital to the environment in which they exist. Each brain hemisphere is subdivided into four lobes, each with specific functions:

- The frontal lobes, situated right behind the forehead, are the brain's center for reasoning, planning, and problem solving. This area controls how you understand language and produce speech. It is also involved in movement, impulse control, emotions, and personality.
- The parietal lobes, just behind the frontal lobes at the center of the skull, are where we perceive and interpret sensory information: touch, pressure, temperature, and pain.
- The temporal lobes, behind the temples at the sides of the forehead, are instrumental to memory and learning. They are also where you recognize sounds.
- The occipital lobes, at the back of each hemisphere, detect and process visual images. This part of the brain is sometimes called the visual cortex.

The Limbic System: The Emotional Brain

Deep within the brain is the limbic system, sometimes called the emotional brain. It links your brain stem and automatic body functions with the more highly evolved intellectual areas of the cerebral cortex. The limbic system consists of several structures:

- The hypothalamus is in charge of homeostasis, or maintaining the body's status quo. It regulates body temperature, hunger, and thirst, and is involved in emotion and your sleep cycle.
- The thalamus serves as a relay station for nearly all sensory information that travels to and from the cerebrum and the rest of the body.
- The amygdala controls memory, emotion, and fear. It triggers the so-called fight-or-flight response.
- The hippocampus is vital to learning and memory, particularly converting your short-term memory into long-term. This part of the brain also helps you comprehend spatial

relationships and navigate the world around you. The hippocampus is one of the first parts of the brain that suffers damage from plaques and tangles in the course of Alzheimer's disease.

📋 Fact

The course Alzheimer's takes depends in part on age at diagnosis and the presence of other conditions that compromise a person's health. Changes may begin twenty years or more before diagnosis. Mild to moderate Alzheimer's generally lasts from two to ten years. Severe Alzheimer's may last from one to five years, according to the Alzheimer's Association.

The Nervous System

Alzheimer's disease disrupts and destroys the brain's ecosystem by devastating what scientists call a neuron forest.

Your brain is made up of an estimated 100 billion specialized nerve cells, or neurons. Each neuron consists of a cell body, one or more specialized branch-like extensions called dendrites (which receive nerve signals), and a single axon (which sends or transmits signals from the cell body to other neurons).

Neurons contain chemicals called *neurotransmitters* that enable cells to communicate across tiny gaps called *synapses*. The tens of billions of neurons in your brain connect at 100 trillion points.

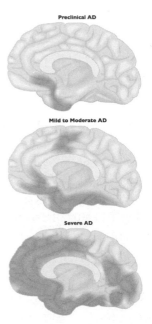

Preclinical AD

Mild to Moderate AD

Severe AD

When a neuron is stimulated, it receives messages from other cells. A tiny impulse, or electrical charge, builds in the cell body and travels to the end of the axon. There, it stimulates tiny sacs that release neurotransmitters to enable communication between nerve cells across a synapse. The typical neuron has up to 15,000 synapses.

Fact

Scientists have discovered unusually low levels of acetylcholine, a neurotransmitter critical to learning and memory, in the brains of people with AD. The neurotransmitters serotonin, norepinephrine, somatostatin, and GABA are depleted in nearly half of people with Alzheimer's. Neurotransmitter imbalance can contribute significantly to insomnia, depression, aggression, and mood swings.

As Alzheimer's disease takes hold in the brain, neurons stop functioning, lose connections with one another, and die. The death of many neurons causes vital parts of the brain to atrophy, devastating your ability to remember, think, and control how your brain and body behave.

How Alzheimer's Disease Affects Memory

Normal aging leads to changes in the brain, especially in areas involved in learning and memory. Some of the neurons shrink; others are damaged over time by molecules called free radicals, which destroy fats and proteins that are essential to normal cell function. High blood pressure or elevated low-density lipoprotein (LDL) cholesterol also take a toll.

Widespread neuron damage isn't normal, but these changes can make it more difficult for an older person to learn new things or to recall information from memory. With Alzheimer's disease, the damage is more severe. Alzheimer's affects different memory systems—episodic, semantic, procedural, and working—in multiple areas of the brain.

⌷. Essential

Neurons do their jobs and communicate through an electrochemical process, a system that controls vital body functions and enables you to see, think, move, talk, remember, and feel emotions. Groups of neurons in your brain have subspecialties: Some are involved with thinking, learning, and memory. Others take in sensory information. Still others send messages to muscles, stimulating them into action.

According to the *Johns Hopkins Memory Bulletin*, Alzheimer's interferes with each memory system:

- Episodic memory enables us to learn new information and remember recent events. The temporal lobe, which contains the hippocampus, and the prefrontal cortex are important to episodic memory, which recovers memories of recent events. The hippocampus is one of the first brain structures damaged in early Alzheimer's, which is why people with AD have difficulty remembering recent events but don't have trouble remembering events from long ago.
- Semantic memory governs general knowledge and facts, including the ability to recognize, name, and categorize things. People with Alzheimer's often have trouble naming common objects (the phone or television) or listing objects that fall within a category (dishes, glasses, and cutlery with which to set a table).
- Procedural memory enables you to learn skills that become automatic, such as typing, skiing, or grooming yourself. This memory system usually isn't damaged until the middle or later stages of the disease.

- Working memory, which governs attention, concentration, and the short-term retention of helpful information, such as a phone number, helps you pay attention and do things that involve multiple steps or tasks. Problems with working memory are characteristic of cognitive disorders, such as Alzheimer's disease, dementia with Lewy bodies, Parkinson's disease, and Huntington's disease.

LEARNING AND ADJUSTING

Joan Cahill knew something was wrong. "I've never been good at directions, but I became really bad at directions," the retired nurse told NurseWeek.com, an online nursing magazine published by the Gannett Healthcare Group. "One time, I got lost en route to my sister-in-law's house—a route I had taken many times. Another time, I found myself in a store that I had shopped at fairly frequently and they had redone their displays, so things were not in the order I remembered them. That episode was very frightening."

At first, Cahill thought her disorientation and confusion might be symptoms of depression. "I had a sister who died after a long illness, and then I had surgery. Not long after that, my brother died in a fire in his home. In the middle of all this, I had a stroke, but I made a good recovery," she explains. "There was also some anxiety around paperwork, bills, and scheduling. This all happened within a fairly short period of time, so surely that figured in.

"My family also was beginning to notice I was repeating myself and having trouble finding the right words. I always have loved words, but was having a difficult time expressing myself."

Living with Alzheimer's means making a series of adjustments, Cahill acknowledges. For her, the hardest was giving up driving. "I hate being dependent on others for rides," she said. She also found that "it generally takes me much longer to do things than in the past. Once able to read a few books a month, it now takes me forever to read just one. Multitasking is exhausting."

She wishes her fellow health care professionals knew a little more and showed a lot more patience and understanding of people with Alzheimer's. "There have been times when I have gone to the doctor's office and been ignored," she said. "The doctors sometimes have to be reminded to talk with me, not just my family."

Early-Stage Alzheimer's Disease

The earliest noticeable signs of Alzheimer's are subtle. They are often mistaken for normal aging or senility. That is particularly true because many people with AD appear to be healthy and functioning normally at home, at work, and in social situations.

Question

What's the difference between early-onset and early-stage Alzheimer's?
The vast majority of people with Alzheimer's are age sixty-five or older. People in this situation are said to have late-onset Alzheimer's. A rare form of the disorder that strikes people between the ages of thirty and sixty-five is called early-onset or young-onset Alzheimer's. Early-stage Alzheimer's describes the first noticeable symptoms of the disease, whether it is late-onset or early-onset.

Destruction of neurons takes hold first in parts of the brain that control memory, especially the hippocampus. That's why memory impairment is often the first sign of Alzheimer's disease. As nerve cells in the hippocampus break down, memory of recent events begins to fail, and the ability to do familiar tasks begins to decline.

SPOTTING EARLY-STAGE ALZHEIMER'S

Disorientation and confusion are common signs of early-stage AD that many people miss, say those who have lived with Alzheimer's.

"My mom couldn't keep track of the time of day or day of the week, and she couldn't keep track of money," says Terry, who lived near his mother and saw her almost daily once she developed Alzheimer's. "She started missing her bridge clubs or lunch with her friends because she got the day wrong. She could cover for it—for a while. But then she really couldn't keep the days straight, and she'd be all dressed and ready to go to somewhere the wrong day or not home when someone came to pick her up."

Terry's mother was living in her own apartment in an elder-care community, and she ate dinner in the dining room there. Otherwise, there was no one to keep track of her comings and goings.

"One time I showed up to take her to one of the kids' ball-games and then go to dinner," recalls Terry. "She wasn't there. I waited an hour, then went to the game, which was about an hour away, and kept calling her.

"I finally got hold of her when the game was over, and she said, 'Why haven't you picked me up for the game?' I explained what happened, and she said she'd been to dinner. Then she asked when I was coming to take her to the game. I explained that the game was over, and she asked me to take her to dinner.

"It turns out, she'd gone to dinner, but she'd gone at the wrong time. So she was hungry. It was nine o'clock at night, and I was an hour away.

"God knows how many times this happened. Probably a lot. It probably contributed to her stomach problems, on top of everything else."

While each person is different, many people with AD experience these symptoms and problems:

- **Memory loss.** She frequently forgets familiar words, names, and recent events. She regularly loses objects (her keys) or leaves them in peculiar places (the fridge).
- **Confusion.** She loses her sense of time, date, and place. She may confuse days of the week or weeks and months on a calendar.
- **Disorientation.** She may get lost in familiar places. This is very frustrating to many people with early-stage AD.
- **Difficulty handling money.** A chaotic checkbook is an early sign of dementia, experts say. She may have trouble with basic math calculations or balancing a checkbook.
- **Trouble concentrating and learning new things.** If she has difficulty following conversations or simple directions (in an exercise class, for example), she may withdraw from new or challenging situations.
- **Poor judgment or decision-making.** She gets bewildered by routine, noncatastrophic problems (like locking herself out of the house) and responds oddly (wandering the neighborhood until she reaches someone by phone). People with early-stage dementia may agree to give away large sums of money. She may be duped by unscrupulous telemarketers and is more likely to become a victim of fraud.
- **Decreased ability to plan and carry out a sequence of actions:** for example, making a doctor's appointment or packing for a trip.
- **She may be restless or anxious.**
- **Mood swings.** Occasional personality changes may occur.

Middle-Stage Alzheimer's

As Alzheimer's progresses, it moves into the cerebral cortex, damaging areas in the temporal, frontal, and parietal lobes responsible for language, reasoning, perception, and judgment. An AD sufferer may find it more and more difficult to express herself and to understand what others are saying.

This is the stage in which many people with AD begin to behave in what seems to be bizarre or inappropriate ways. Increasingly confused by the world around her, her judgment diminished, a person with AD may be prone to emotional outbursts. She may be restless and agitated, particularly late in the day. Individuals with mid-stage AD may experience these symptoms:

- **Increased memory loss.** Forgetfulness begins to interfere with daily activity. She has some problems recognizing friends and family and may not recall her own address and phone number. She forgets key events in her own life. Because memories are so important to the human sense of self, she begins to lose self-awareness.
- **Difficulty performing basic tasks like making tea or coffee.** She may be overwhelmed by household chores.
- **Confusion.** Increasingly disconnected from the world around her, she forgets current events in the world at large and her own life. She may think a show on TV is real, and confuse a plot with her own life.
- **Shortened attention span.** She has difficulty reading, writing, and doing basic math.
- **Communication problems.** She has trouble following conversations, and in gathering and expressing thoughts.
- **Visual-spatial disorientation.** Many people with AD lose their sense of geography, spatial relations, and where their bodies are in relation to the physical world. She may be

uncoordinated and awkward. She may have trouble setting a table or getting in and out of a car.

- **Loss of impulse control.** She may curse, swear, and forget her table manners. She might refuse to dress appropriately either for an occasion or the weather and may undress spontaneously or even masturbate in public. She may behave amorously toward someone other than her spouse or mistake a stranger for her husband.
- **Anxiety and fearfulness.**
- **Restlessness, pacing, and repetitive movements such as hand wringing and tissue shredding.**
- **Hallucinations.** A hallucination is a mistaken sensory perception of objects or events that seem real to a person but are not actually happening. The most common hallucinations are visual (seeing something that isn't there) and auditory (hearing something that isn't there), but taste, smell, and touch may also be involved.
- **Delusions, depression, and agitation.** A delusion is a false or peculiar conviction a person firmly believes despite overwhelming evidence to the contrary. Common delusions among dementia patients involve suspicion—that people are hiding things or stealing from them—or that a spouse is having an affair.
- **Disrupted sleep cycle.** She may take naps during the day and be active from late afternoon through the night.

Severe and Late-Stage Alzheimer's

In the later stages of Alzheimer's, the patient's cognitive abilities devolve dramatically. Personality changes and idiosyncratic behavior become extreme. The brain loses control of the body; and the physical symptoms of illness are profound.

In late-stage Alzheimer's, you may see the following symptoms in your loved one:

- Inability to recognize family.
- Inability to perform activities of daily living (e.g., bathing, toileting, eating).
- Loss of awareness of surroundings.
- Declining ability to speak.
- Inability to walk without help or sit without support.
- Inability to hold up head.
- Loss of ability to smile.
- Can't write or comprehend writing.
- Bedridden.
- Can't swallow easily and may choke on her food.
- Prone to infections.
- May have seizures.
- Sleeps continually.
- Sensory organs shut down.

Source: *National Institute on Aging*

As the end of life approaches, Alzheimer's patients are utterly helpless. Most need round-the-clock care. Family and caregivers will have to decide where it is possible—and preferable—for her to receive that care. Doctors, nurses, and hospice care providers can help you make these decisions.

CHAPTER 3

Making Sure
It's Alzheimer's

A mericans over age fifty-five fear Alzheimer's more than cancer, according to a 2006 report by the MetLife Foundation.
Unfortunately, that dread discourages far too many people from
seeking medical diagnosis of memory loss and cognitive problems
that may or may not indicate AD. Alzheimer's, vascular dementia,
and Lewy body dementia are progressive, irreversible diseases, but
symptoms can be treated. And some causes of dementia—thyroid
gland problems, dehydration, vitamin deficiency, or medication
side effects—can be treated and sometimes reversed.

The Importance of Early Diagnosis

Surveys show that many people who care for those with clear signs
of memory loss often wait two to three years before seeking a diagnosis of the condition. Some well-intentioned caregivers may think
they're protecting a loved one from worry or depression by delaying
a dismal diagnosis. Others worry that receiving a diagnosis would
be a self-fulfilling prophecy and somehow worsen symptoms of the
disease. But ignorance is by no means bliss. In fact, living with undiagnosed memory loss, chronic confusion, and other symptoms of
dementia is worrisome, distressing, and frequently depressing, say
many people who've had the experience.

Delaying diagnosis can make it more difficult to treat symptoms of any condition or disease. Medications that are available

to treat symptoms of Alzheimer's and other degenerative brain diseases usually work best in early stages of the disease. And while those drugs don't halt the course of the illness, they are known to improve the quality of life for some patients and caregivers. And that, in turn, can delay the need for assisted living or admission to a nursing home.

What Is Dementia?

Dementia itself is not a disease but a term that describes different brain disorders that cause memory loss and other symptoms of cognitive decline. While various kinds of dementia are more common the longer we live, none is a part of normal aging. Dementia specialists recommend you see a doctor to evaluate any of these problems or symptoms, which may point to dementia:

- Problems retaining recent memories and learning new information, losing and misplacing objects, regularly forgetting appointments or recent conversations, or asking the same question over and over.
- Problems handling complex tasks; trouble balancing a checkbook, following a recipe, or performing routine tasks that involve a complex train of thought.
- Trouble reasoning. Difficulty dealing with everyday problems, such as a flat tire. Uncharacteristic rash behavior, including poor financial or social judgment.
- Difficulty with spatial ability and orientation. Driving and navigating familiar surroundings becomes difficult; trouble recognizing local landmarks.
- Difficulty with language. Problems speaking, listening, and following or participating in conversations.
- Behavioral or personality changes. An active, engaged person seems listless and unresponsive. Trusting people become suspicious.

Irreversible Dementias

Alzheimer's, vascular dementia, and Lewy body dementia are the most common irreversible dementias. Frontotemporal dementia, mixed dementia, and dementias that develop with Parkinson's disease, Huntington's disease, and rare, infectious diseases (such as Creutzfeldt-Jakob disease) are also incurable. However, drugs and other treatments can help reduce some symptoms of these disorders.

Vascular Dementia

Vascular dementia (sometimes called multi-infarct dementia), which accounts for 10 to 20 percent of all dementia cases, is cognitive impairment caused by reduced blood flow to the brain. It is usually caused by strokes that interrupt normal blood flow, destroying brain cells and brain functions. Vascular dementia can also result from lupus and other autoimmune inflammatory diseases. In some cases of vascular dementia, a major stroke strikes suddenly and severely, bringing on a sudden loss of cognitive function.

 Alert

Older adults take an average of more than five prescription drugs and three over-the-counter drugs at the same time, say experts at Johns Hopkins University Medical School. In geriatric clinics, an adverse reaction to medications is the most common cause of reversible dementia.

More often, the disease is caused by a series of transient ischemic attacks (TIAs) or mini-strokes, whose symptoms may last just a few minutes and usually subside within an hour. Individually, these strokes don't do much damage. But the cumulative effect of multiple, recurring TIAs can destroy enough brain tissue to impair memory, reasoning, language, and other cognitive abilities, specialists say.

According to the National Institute of Neurological Disorders and Stroke (NINDS), you should watch for these stroke symptoms:

- Sudden confusion, trouble speaking, or trouble understanding speech
- Sudden trouble seeing in one or both eyes
- Sudden trouble walking, dizziness, loss of balance or coordination
- Sudden severe headache with no known cause

Symptoms of vascular dementia often resemble those brought on by heart attack or stroke: confusion, depression, loss of bladder or bowel control, and unsteadiness. The cognitive symptoms may appear in steps, with a gradual loss in thinking and impaired executive functions, such as planning and completing tasks.

Essential

A transient ischemic attack (TIA), or mini-stroke, is no minor matter. TIA symptoms usually subside in less than an hour. But TIAs are medical emergencies that should be diagnosed and treated within an hour, according to the National Institute of Neurological Disorders and Stroke. Transient strokes are often warning signs of more debilitating strokes in the future.

Many people with vascular dementia suffer from chronic high blood pressure, diabetes, or coronary heart disease (a narrowing of the coronary arteries that reduces blood flow to the heart). Doctors can sometimes slow or even halt progression of the dementia by treating those underlying conditions.

Mixed Dementia

Brain autopsies in recent years have revealed that as many as 45 percent of people with dementia have signs of both Alzheimer's and vascular dementia. The presence of both diseases is more common than experts once believed and seems to occur more frequently in patients of advanced age. People with mixed dementia may have symptoms of AD, vascular dementia, or both. The combined disorders may cause more problematic symptoms than either by itself.

Lewy Body Dementia

You may never have heard of Lewy body dementia (LBD), even though it is the second most common neurodegenerative dementia in older people. Sometimes referred to as Lewy body disease, dementia with Lewy bodies, or diffuse Lewy body disease, LBD is poorly understood and often misdiagnosed, in part because it shares some characteristics of both Alzheimer's and Parkinson's disease.

Like Alzheimer's, LBD impairs thinking and memory. Like Parkinson's, it can cause muscle stiffness, problems moving and walking, listlessness, and apathy. The disease appears to be caused by Lewy bodies, spherical deposits of a protein called alpha-synuclein, which develop in and destroy regions of the brain responsible for thinking and movement.

Lewy body symptoms are distinct, particularly in the early stages. People with Lewy body dementia are more prone to problems with executive function, such as organizing and planning, and spatial orientation, such as physical awkwardness and getting lost, than with memory loss.

Rather than following a progressive, predictable pattern, symptoms fluctuate. A majority of people with LBD go in and out of periods of alertness and confusion. This can happen from day to day, hour to hour, even minute to minute, making detection and diagnosis difficult.

An estimated 80 percent of LBD patients have vivid, colorful, three-dimensional visual hallucinations, particularly at night, specialists say. These hallucinations are not particularly distressing to the patient, who may also experience daytime hallucinations (thinking someone is present who isn't, for example).

LBD sufferers are also particularly prone to depression, sleep disturbance, daytime drowsiness, staring into space, and disorganized speech.

Alert

As many as 50 percent of patients with Lewy body are acutely sensitive to medications sometimes prescribed to treat hallucinations and other psychiatric disorders. Traditional antipsychotic medications such as haloperidol (Haldol), fluphenazine (Prolixin), and chlorpromazine (Thorazine), can set off severe reactions in people with Lewy body disease.

Experts stress the importance of an accurate diagnosis in treating people with Lewy body disease and urge caution in prescribing AD drugs to Lewy body patients. Some patients respond to cholinesterase inhibitors, which can help improve alertness and cognition and may help reduce hallucinations and other behavioral problems. But Parkinson's disease medications that are sometimes prescribed to help reduce Parkinson's-like muscular symptoms can worsen dementia symptoms in people with LBD.

WHAT I WISH I'D KNOWN ABOUT LEWY BODY

"Toward the end of my mother's life, it became clear she'd been suffering not from Alzheimer's, as everyone assumed, but dementia with Lewy bodies. I mentioned this to her doctor, who basically brushed it off and said they had a limited number of drugs for people with all late-stage dementias and they treated all of them the same," says Elizabeth.

"The trouble is, Lewy body might end up the same as Alzheimer's. But it doesn't begin the same way and doesn't have the same symptoms as Alzheimer's does. And in my mother's case, knowing that could have made a difference in the quality of the last year or so of her life, and it could have saved her some pain.

"I wish we'd known, for example, that getting lost all the time—in her own neighborhood or driving home from one of our houses to hers—was an early sign of Lewy body disease. This was a woman who had a terrific sense of direction."

Elizabeth regrets not knowing about characteristic Lewy body symptoms. "I wish I'd known why this person who handled money well all her life was suddenly losing cash everywhere she went. Or why this incredible conversationalist was all of a sudden interrupting people when they were talking, or staring into space and losing track of what she was saying. I wish we'd known that people with this disease go in and out of it, that there were reasons she was sleeping all the time, and why she seemed to have all this acute back and muscle pain!" she says.

"I *really* wish the doctors in her assisted living and long-term care facilities had known she had Lewy body disease. If they had, they might not have given her anti-psychotics—which made her nuts—and they might have paid more attention to her physical pain, which made her very unhappy in the last year of her life. Doctors ought to know at least not to take a one-size-fits-all approach to dementia, the disease."

Frontotemporal Dementia

Frontotemporal dementias (FTD) are a group of degenerative brain diseases that attack the frontal and temporal lobes. Those parts of the brain control judgment, personality, movement, speech, language, social awareness, and some elements of memory. Characteristic symptoms of FTD include antisocial or inappropriate behavior, such as stealing, reckless spending, or making rude or off-color remarks. Those symptoms, which frequently emerge between ages forty and sixty-five, are sometimes misdiagnosed and treated as psychological or emotional problems.

Pick's disease, which is thought to account for approximately one-third of frontotemporal dementia cases, is characterized by problems with language, loss of social skills, and personality changes that usually appear in middle age and get worse with time. People with Pick's disease are often not aware their symptoms are problematic, specialists say. Other neurological diseases associated with dementia—corticobasal ganglionic degeneration, motor neuron disease–inclusion dementia, primary progressive aphasia, and progressive supranuclear palsy—may involve abnormalities similar to those associated with frontotemporal dementia, researchers say.

Other Degenerative Diseases Associated with Dementia

Three devastating diseases, Parkinson's disease, Huntington's disease, and Creutzfeldt-Jakob disease, can cause irreversible dementia.

Parkinson's Disease

Parkinson's attacks nerve cells, or neurons, in the part of the brain that controls muscle movement. It damages neurons that make dopamine, a neurotransmitter that normally sends signals that help coordinate movement and balance. As neurons deteriorate and die off, people with Parkinson's develop stiffness in their arms, legs, and trunk; problems with movement; and poor balance and coordination. Their hands, arms, legs, and faces may tremble.

Huntington's Disease (HD)

Huntington's causes cell degeneration throughout the brain and spinal cord. People with HD are born with a defective gene, though their symptoms, which include problems with balance, mild personality change, and cognition, don't begin until middle age. HD can cause involuntary jerky movements, muscle weakness, and clumsiness. Gradually, it can take away the ability to walk, talk, or swallow. People with Huntington's often develop dementia in later stages of the disease.

▤ Fact

People with severe Parkinson's may develop dementia-like symptoms, which can also be a side effect of some of the medications used to treat the disorder. Side effects of Levodopa, considered the most effective Parkinson's drug, for example, include confusion, delusions, and hallucinations as well as dyskinesia (involuntary movements).

Creutzfeldt-Jakob Disease (CJD)

Creutzfeldt-Jakob disease (pronounced CROYZ-felt YAH-cob) is a very rare, fast-moving, and fatal brain disease that each year strikes approximately 1 out of 1 million people worldwide, including 200 people living in the United States. CJD is the most common known human form of a family of diseases called *transmissible spongiform encephalopathies*. During the 1990s, a new variety of CJD, variant Creutzfeldt-Jakob disease (vCJD), which is believed to be caused by eating meat from cattle affected by mad cow disease, was identified in humans. CJD is very difficult to diagnose; its many symptoms include signs of dementia as well as general changes in well-being such as sleep problems, headaches, and appetite loss.

Treatable Causes of Dementia

Endocrine abnormalities, metabolic disturbances, nutritional deficiencies, infections, AIDS, traumatic brain injury, and a certain form of hydrocephalus can cause or mimic dementia. Get an early, accurate diagnosis of symptoms to help a doctor make a diagnosis. Following is a brief explanation of each:

- **Endocrine abnormalities.** High or low thyroid levels and adrenal abnormalities can cause dementia-like confusion.
- **Metabolic disorders.** Confusion and changes in sleep, appetite, and emotional state may be signs of hypoglycemia (low blood sugar), electrolyte imbalances, or kidney or liver failure.
- **Nutritional deficiencies.** Dehydration, common in older adults, can cause confusion. Deficiencies of B vitamins (folate, niacin, riboflavin, and thiamine) are strongly associated with cognitive impairment.
- **Infections.** Encephalitis, an inflammation of the brain that causes irritation and swelling, and meningitis, which inflames membranes that cover the brain and spinal cord, can spur memory loss or sudden dementia. Infectious diseases including syphilis can do the same.
- **AIDS** (acquired immune deficiency syndrome). AIDS, which occurs in the most advanced stages of human immunodeficiency virus (HIV) infection, is an immune system disorder that also damages the nervous system. It can cause brain inflammation, producing confusion, forgetfulness, and behavioral changes. AIDS-dementia complex (ADC) or HIV-associated encephalopathy usually occur with more advanced HIV infection, causing symptoms that include encephalitis, behavioral changes, and a gradual decline in cognitive function. Left untreated, ADC can be fatal.
- **Traumatic brain injury.** A blow to the head, a fall, an automobile accident, or anything else that traumatizes the brain can damage or destroy brain cells, resulting in symptoms of dementia such as behavioral changes, memory loss, confusion, disorientation, and other cognitive problems.
- **Normal pressure hydrocephalus** (NPH). This form of hydrocephalus occurs when excess fluid surrounding the brain and spinal cord cannot drain normally. As fluid builds up,

the ventricles (fluid-filled chambers) inside the brain expand, compressing and damaging nearby tissue. Certain kinds of head injuries, infections such as meningitis, and bleeding inside the brain can cause NPH.

THE NFL AND ALZHEIMER'S

Retired National Football League players face a 37 percent higher risk of Alzheimer's than other males of the same age in the United States, according to a 2007 University of North Carolina study.

Most people know that severe blows to the head are bad. Studies of boxers show that at least 20 percent of people who suffer repeated brain trauma go on to develop degenerative brain disease, according Dr. Ann McKee at Boston University's Center for the Study of Traumatic Encephalopathy. But few suspected that football players who suffer repeated concussions during their playing days are at higher risk for depression, mild cognitive impairment, and Alzheimer's.

Evidently, they are.

McKee, who has studied the brains of several former NFL players who died before they turned fifty, says the players' brains have sustained damage similar to what she sees in some aging boxers. Their brain cells had shrunk, and tangles (a hallmark of dementia) had started to appear.

"You don't see anything like this in the normal population," McKee told National Public Radio.

Damage from traumatic brain injuries may not appear for years after a player starts playing. But, she says, "once it's triggered, it just keeps on progressing." And that can lead to memory deficits, depression, and, eventually, dementia.

McKee says it's likely that some players carry genes that make them more vulnerable to head injuries. (The ApoE4 allele is thought to make some people extremely sensitive to the effects of traumatic brain injury.)

She hopes to learn more by studying at least 100 brains from former football players—research that could take years, since she can only study brains of players who agree before they die to donate their brains to science.

Distinguishing Delirium and Dementia

Delirium is not the same thing as dementia. It's a sudden change in mental function—a state of acute confusion and agitation. It is one of the most common complications of medical illness or recovery from surgery among older adults in the hospital.

Fact

One-third of older adults arriving at hospital emergency departments are delirious, and approximately one-third of patients age seventy or older who are admitted to the hospital for general medical care experience delirium while they are there. Delirium is even more common among older adults admitted to intensive care units. Delirium occurs in half of hospital patients transferred to nursing homes.

The American Geriatrics Society has published symptoms that characterize and distinguish symptoms of both disorders:

DEMENTIA
- Slow onset over months to years
- Normal speech
- Conscious and attentive
- Memory loss
- Language difficulties
- Hallucinations possible
- Listless or apathetic mood; agitation also possible
- Often no other signs of illness

DELIRIUM
- Sudden onset over hours to days
- Slurred speech
- In and out of consciousness; inattentive, easily distracted
- Memory loss
- Hallucinations common
- May be anxious, fearful, suspicious, or agitated—or apathetic
- Signs of medical illness such as fever or chills; drug side effects

Is It Dementia or Depression?

Memory problems, confusion, and a loss of interest in things that normally give you pleasure are among the warning signs of dementia. These are also symptoms of clinical depression, a debilitating, often undiagnosed disorder that strikes as many as 17 million American adults each year.

Essential

If you've lived through bouts of depression, you may recognize its symptoms when they occur. Depression can cause feelings of hopelessness or helplessness. It can also appear as anger and discouragement. Severe depression can even cause hallucinations and delusions. If you or a loved one is depressed, consult with a health professional.

Depression is not a normal part of aging. It's a treatable illness caused by a chemical imbalance that affects some 15 percent of adults over age sixty-five at some point. Retirement, health problems, loss of friends and loved ones, and concerns about mortality are part and parcel of older adulthood. A sense of sadness is normal at times. But persistent sadness that saps your energy and interest in life can signal a problem.

Dementia as a Side Effect
of Prescription Drugs

Older adults, who make up 13 percent of the population, consume 30 percent of prescription drugs. Many commonly prescribed medications cause cognitive problems, not only among older patients with dementia, but among those with no existing impairment, according to Peter V. Rabins, MD, director of geriatrics and neuropsychiatry at Johns Hopkins University.

 Alert

> Remember, medications can affect you differently at age sixty than they did when you were forty-five, particularly if you take more than one drug at the same time. Your kidneys may not remove drugs from your bloodstream as quickly; drug metabolism in your liver may slow; and changes in your fat-to-muscle ration increase the time it takes to eliminate some drugs from the body.

Geriatricians and pharmacists warn patients to be wary of anticholinergic medications, a category that includes antihistamines for allergies, anti-anxiety drugs like Xanax, and medications prescribed to prevent heart failure (Lanoxin and Lasix). Anticholinergics can put people at risk for cognitive impairment because they block the neurotransmitter acetylcholine, a chemical brain messenger that stimulates memory and learning, says Dr. Rabins.

Anti-anxiety drugs including Halcion (triazolam) and Xanax can impair memory. The benzodiazepines diazepam (Valium) and lorazepam (Ativan), often prescribed as sedatives and sleeping pills, can cause memory problems in otherwise healthy people—and set off rapid cognitive decline among those with AD, Dr. Rabins warns.

The anti-inflammatory drug prednisone (Deltasone) and heartburn drugs such as Tagamet (cimetidine), Pepcid (famotidine), and Zantac (ranitidine) can also cause memory problems. Antipsychotic drugs like olanzapine (Zyprexa) and aripiprazole

(Abilify), frequently prescribed to treat dementia symptoms of agitation and aggression, exacerbate dementia symptoms in some patients, according to Dr. Rabins.

Essential

Someone who's being evaluated for dementia may not be able to recall accurately when, how, and in what order his symptoms emerged. He may underestimate the problem. It's important that a caregiver, family member, or friend who knows the patient well accompany him to the evaluation and provide this information to the doctor or nurse.

Many medications can interact with drugs used to treat Alzheimer's and other dementias, including Aricept, Exelon, and Razadyne, according to federal health officials. Some over-the-counter medications, including cough and cold remedies and sleep medicines, may also react with other medications taken by someone with AD. Indeed, some people with cognitive impairment caused by medication may be prescribed a drug like donepezil (Aricept)—which is a procholinergic Alzheimer's medication—to counteract the effects of the anticholinergic drug they are taking. Treat yourself sensibly: Consult a health professional before using prescription or over-the-counter medications.

THE DIFFICULTY OF DIAGNOSING ALZHEIMER'S

Most diagnoses of Alzheimer's are delayed until more than two years after symptoms first appear because patients and families ignore, deny, or don't recognize common signs of early Alzheimer's, according to a 2006 Alzheimer's Foundation of America survey. Fifty-seven percent of caregivers who answered the poll said they put off seeking diagnosis for symptoms of memory loss, confusion, and language difficulties because they—or the person they cared for—were in denial about having the disease, or because they feared the social stigma associated with AD. Another 40 percent didn't seek a diagnosis because they knew little about Alzheimer's or its symptoms, they said.

38 percent of those surveyed said it was the patient who resisted going to see a doctor; 19 percent of caregivers admitted they themselves didn't want to face the possibility that something was wrong. Spouses were three times less likely than children of people with Alzheimer's to delay seeking diagnosis, the survey found.

Diagnosing Dementia

If a health professional suspects a serious cognitive problem, you should undergo a thorough medical and neuropsychological evaluation. That will help determine what is causing dementia symptoms and how to treat them. A dementia diagnosis will most likely include many of the following steps and procedures:

- **Description of the history or sudden onset of symptoms.** You or your loved one may be asked to describe problems in detail: In what order did things happen? How long have the symptoms been present? How do they affect the patient's daily life?
- **Review of medical history and medications.** This information can help identify other conditions that may be causing symptoms and indicate a patient's risk for a particular type of dementia or disease. It can help identify side effects from medications that may contribute to or even be causing the problems. Be sure to bring medications—or at least an accurate list of drugs and doses—to the appontment.
- **Physical examination.** A physical exam helps rule out treatable causes of dementia and identifies signs of stroke or other illnesses, such as heart disease or kidney failure.
- **Neurological evaluations.** A neurological examination looks at balance, sensory function, reflexes, and other functions

to identify signs of conditions such as movement disorders or stroke that may cause or contribute to symptoms.

- **Cognitive and neuropsychological tests.** These tests measure memory, language skills, math skills, and other signs of mental functioning, such as problem solving. Doctors often use a test called the Mini Mental State Examination (MMSE) to assess cognitive skills in people with suspected dementia, although the MMSE cannot be used alone to diagnose Alzheimer's disease.
- **Laboratory tests to rule out vitamin deficiencies or metabolic conditions.** Occasionally, a simple vitamin deficiency, infection, or hormone imbalance can cause cognitive symptoms. Some laboratory tests may indicate a condition that puts a person at risk for developing dementia, such as high cholesterol or high blood pressure.
- **Imaging techniques.** Doctors may use imaging techniques to identify strokes, tumors, or other problems that can cause dementia. The most common types of brain scans are computed tomographic (CT) scans, magnetic resonance imaging (MRI), and positron emission tomography (PET).

The process of diagnosing dementia has become more accurate in recent years, and specialists are able to collect and analyze a range of indicators to determine whether and why a problem may exist, and how it should be treated.

CHAPTER 4

The New Normal: How Your Body, Brain, and Memory Change with Age

Not too long ago, physical frailty and chronic memory loss were considered natural signs of older age. Physicians knew very little about normal, healthy aging because relatively few people lived past age sixty-five. Average life expectancy in the United States was forty-seven years in 1900. By 2005, it had risen to seventy-eight. Today, more than 13 percent of Americans are sixty-five and older, and their ranks are growing as baby boomers age. Seniors and soon-to-be seniors expect to live longer, healthier, and more active lives.

Normal Physical Aging: The Basics

You can't have a healthy brain without a healthy body. And you're more likely to enjoy both if you know what to expect and what could be cause for concern as you age.

None of us ages at the same pace, of course. But if you live to a ripe old age, it's inevitable you will lose some—though by no means all—of your physical strength and speed.

Your body and brain achieve their peak function shortly before you turn thirty and then begin a slow, steady decline. Most changes occur slowly over a number of years and are barely noticeable.

You age because your cells—the basic units of life and the building blocks of all the tissues and organs in your body—grow older. They become less efficient at reproducing, receiving oxygen and nutrients, and eliminating carbon dioxide and toxic wastes. Some begin to function abnormally. Some die off.

Gradually, the capacity of your heart, brain, kidneys, and other organs declines. Few people notice this, because human organs have more functional capacity than we ever need. That reserve is what allows your body to function with a single kidney, and your brain to reshape and redirect itself if you suffer a head injury. After age thirty, you lose an average of 1 percent of this reserve each year.

Most of your organs should function adequately throughout your lifetime, unless they're attacked by disease, injury, environmental factors, or what doctors call lifestyle behaviors such as cigarette smoking, alcoholism, or poor diet. Any and all of those stressors can force organs to work harder, diminishing their functional reserve. A decline in one organ's function frequently affects others, straining vital organs and systems.

Normal Changes in Your Musculoskeletal System

If you've been fairly healthy most of your life, you may be surprised to wake up one morning with muscle aches and pains. Most people feel the first effects of age in the musculoskeletal system.

Bones and Joints

In middle age, your bones lose calcium and other minerals. They get thinner and weaker and are more inclined to break. Bones in your hips, wrists, and spine weaken more than others. Many women lose bone density rapidly after menopause because their bodies produce less estrogen, which helps strengthen bones.

The cartilage that lines your joints also tends to thin from years of wear and tear. Damage to the cartilage from overuse or repeated injury often leads to osteoarthritis, one of the most common physical afflictions of later life. Between the ages of forty and fifty, osteoarthritis is more prevalent in women than men; middle-aged men usually don't have arthritis, unless it's caused by an earlier trauma from an accident or sports injury. Men in their seventies and eighties, however, develop osteoarthritis as often as women do.

Question

Is it possible to get shorter as you age?
Yes, you can get shorter as you get older. Vertebrae in your spine lose density as you age. The disks, gel-like cushions between each bone, lose fluid and become thinner. The spinal column curves and compresses. Your spine and trunk get shorter, and so do you.

Ligaments, which bind joints together, and tendons that bind your muscles to bones tend to become less elastic, making joints feel tight or stiff. You become less flexible. Ligaments tend to tear more easily and heal more slowly as you get older.

Muscles and Fat

By your seventy-fifth birthday, the percentage of muscle mass in your body is approximately half what it was when you turned twenty-five. Meanwhile, the proportion made up of fat has doubled and is redistributed in your body, which changes shape.

Muscle changes often begin in men while they're in their twenties and in women during their forties. In general, you start losing muscle mass when you're about thirty and continue to do so throughout life. Too much body fat can increase the risk of health problems, including heart disease and diabetes. It can change the way you metabolize foods and medications. It can strain your muscles and bones and limit your mobility.

Most older people retain enough muscle mass and strength to do most physical things they've done throughout adult life. Those who exercise regularly to strengthen muscles can delay or prevent muscle mass loss and avoid some illnesses and injury. Some people remain athletic, compete in sports, and enjoy vigorous activity. But even the fittest experience some decline with age.

Normal Cardiovascular System Changes

As you get older, your heart gets slightly larger. Its wall thickens, and it may pump less blood. The aorta, the main artery from your heart, gets thicker and stiffer, and your other arteries thicken too. As tissues in your blood vessels become less elastic, your blood pressure goes up.

More than half of Americans over age sixty have high blood pressure. However, that does not mean it is part of normal aging, warns the National Institute on Aging. Blood pressure changes all the time depending on physical activity, your emotional state, diet, medication, and whether you're standing, sitting, or lying down.

As you age, you breathe in a little less oxygen. Your lungs lose elasticity and some of their function, and you're more vulnerable to some infections. The muscles you use when you breathe tend to weaken. Exercising and breathing at high altitudes, where there's less oxygen, may get harder. But if you don't smoke or don't suffer from lung damage or disease, you probably won't notice significant changes in the way you breathe during most day-to-day activities.

Normal Changes in the Senses

The way you touch, see, hear, smell, and taste the world changes as you age.

Skin

Your body's largest organ becomes thinner, drier, and more vulnerable with age. Sunlight causes most of the changes we associate with aging, including wrinkles, dryness, and age spots. The fat layer underneath the skin, a cushion and protector that helps keep skin supple and preserves body heat, gets thinner. Your skin looks less plump and smooth. Underlying veins and bones become more prominent. Your skin can take longer to heal. Because you sweat less, your skin gets drier. It may feel flaky or painful.

"Thin" skin makes it harder to adjust to hot and cold temperatures. While your normal body temperature doesn't change significantly in later life, you may find you feel the heat and cold more acutely. Older people are at greater risk for overheating (hyperthermia or heat stroke) and for dangerous drops in body temperature (hypothermia).

Eyes

Whether you've worn glasses since primary school or could always read the smallest print on your eye doctor's chart with ease, you'll find some time after you turn forty that you can't read a road map unless you hold it at arm's length. You'll squint to decipher restaurant menus. You'll switch on lights as you enter rooms and warn your young adult children about the dangers of reading or text messaging in the dark.

Fact

Older people often have trouble deciphering what's said because aging ears lose some ability to clearly hear high-pitched sounds. Consonants (such as k, t, s, and p) are higher-pitched than vowels (a, e, i, o, and u), so it may be difficult to hear high-pitched sounds such as "s" and "th" and tell them apart.

These unmistakable signs of normal aging occur as the lenses of your eyes begin to stiffen and the lens changes shape to help the eye focus. That causes difficulty focusing at near distances, and most people eventually need glasses for reading and close work. Meanwhile, the lens gets denser and cloudier. Less light enters your eyes, and cells of the retina that sense light become less sensitive. That's why it becomes more and more difficult to see in dim light.

On average, a sixty-year-old needs three times more light to read than does a twenty-year-old.

Hearing

If you spend time around teenagers and young adults, you probably know that people over thirty don't hear the high frequency sounds that drive young people crazy. Your ability to hear high-pitched sounds and to distinguish certain sounds gets progressively more difficult as you grow older, thanks to age-related hearing loss.

One in three people age sixty-five and older and about half over seventy-five have trouble hearing normal speech and understanding conversations, particularly if there is background noise. Many develop increased sensitivity to loud noises. Tinnitus—a ringing, roaring, or hissing sound—is not an uncommon complaint.

Taste and Smell

As you age, many of your taste buds disappear. Those that don't go away get duller. Your nose lining gets thinner and drier, its nerve endings disappear, and you can't smell as well.

To compensate for the sensory loss of tantalizing taste and smells, many American adults have grown fond of the intense flavors of spicy food. Mouth-burning, sinus-clearing foods from Mexico and Southeast Asia and Sichuan China, among other places, have grown wildly popular for a variety of reasons, including immigration, globalization, and our increasingly sophisticated national palate. But some of the growth in the hot, spicy food market is merely meeting American baby boomers' demand, say food industry observers. As boomers' natural sense of taste and smell declines, they compensate in other ways.

Changes in the Brain as We Age

Until recently, doctors regularly diagnosed retirees with a catchall condition called *senile dementia*. Senility, as defined in the dictionary, means old age. Physical and mental deterioration were presumed to be part and parcel of the condition. Some of that thinking was based on scientific beliefs about the human brain that have only recently changed.

Until the late twentieth century, scientists thought humans were born with all brain cells already formed, and that brain deterioration was normal as cells died off in large numbers late in life. The brain was thought to be hard-wired once it was fully developed, in late adolescence. Scientists have since learned that brain plasticity continues through adulthood and that it enhances cognitive reserve.

Fact

Massive neuron loss only occurs when the brain is assaulted by trauma, a brain-destroying condition such as stroke, or a neurodegenerative condition such as Alzheimer's disease. The brain has the functional capacity to repair and "rewire" itself.

Stunning scientific discoveries during the 1990s showed that neurons can divide, propagate, and develop into functional new nerve cells in the brain. This process, called *neurogenesis*, is known to occur in the hippocampus (a center of learning and memory) and in a part of the brain involved with smell. This understanding has led to a radical rethinking of the function and dysfunction of the adult human brain.

Your brain reaches its maximum weight when you're about twenty years old and slowly loses about 10 percent of its heft over your lifetime. That happens because neurons shrink, and synapses— the connections between neurons—gradually deteriorate. The brain's supply of neurotransmitters, or chemical messengers, diminishes and communication slows, impeding your ability to think, remember, and calculate quickly. In most cases, these changes are a mere nuisance. They don't interfere with your ability to function from day to day.

Normal Brain Changes: A Timeline

Like the rest of your body, your brain goes through predictable changes over time. Memory experts at Johns Hopkins University Medical School have developed a timeline of how the normal brain ages, which is adapted here.

Question

What is brain plasticity, exactly?
Plasticity is the ability to be formed or molded. Brain plasticity is the brain's ability to adapt to deficits and injury. According to the National Institute of Neurological Disorders and Stroke, "The plasticity of the brain and the rewiring of neural connections make it possible for one part of the brain to take up the functions of a disabled part."

Your Twenties

Between the ages of twenty and thirty, you're typically at the top of your mental game. Your memory is sharp, whether you're recalling details of your childhood, a complicated project, or what you and your friends talked about late last Friday night. Your reasoning skills are strong, and your creativity may be at its peak. Normal neuron shrinkage causes minor physical changes in your brain.

Your Thirties

A battery of cognitive tests might show slight declines from a decade earlier, but most changes are so minor that neither you nor anyone else will notice. Normal neuron shrinkage continues, as your brain slowly loses its volume.

Your Forties

You may sense some slowing of your mental processing, especially in the area of short-term memory. Your slow loss of brain volume continues and may begin to accelerate.

Your memory for phone numbers might get a little fuzzy when you're in your forties. Calculating tips or playing challenging card games may not be quite as easy as they were.

Your Fifties

You cross a threshold in the years between fifty and sixty, a time of accelerated brain volume loss and more noticeable changes in memory, thinking, and learning. Most people need more time to recall names and words and to learn something new. Multitasking gets harder, and your attention to detail wanes. You may find, too, that placing an event in time and place becomes more difficult. You may remember a phone conversation but not when or where you were when you had it, for example. Visual-spatial processing—how easily you can finish jigsaw puzzles or retrace your steps in an unfamiliar place—may get harder.

Your Sixties

The cognitive changes that began in your fifties become more noticeable. It might get harder to concentrate, learn new information, or master complex mental tasks. Your brain has to work harder to form new memories and to recall names, dates, and words. Loss of brain volume continues. Brain structures that are critical to memory and other cognitive abilities may have shrunk by as much as 25 percent.

Your Seventies and Beyond

People in their seventies and eighties vary widely in their cognitive abilities. You may stay quite sharp throughout these years, gaining perspective—even wisdom. This is also an age at which body stressors—high blood pressure, diabetes, smoking, and heavy drinking—will have taken a toll on your memory and general cognitive ability. People who develop dementia typically begin to show signs of the disorder in their mid- to late seventies. Normal memory loss is frustrating but doesn't diminish your day-to-day functioning. With Alzheimer's, memory loss is incapacitating.

Mild Cognitive Impairment

Memory loss specialists have identified a third category of cognitive decline that doesn't fit within the definition of normal age-related memory loss or early-stage Alzheimer's. It's somewhere in between.

What Is MCI?

Mild cognitive impairment (MCI) is a subtle but noticeable disorder that may or may not lead to Alzheimer's. People with MCI have memory impairment that's measurably worse than what's considered normal for people their age. But they show no other signs of early AD and usually function normally at work and in social situations.

 Alert

Age and gender seem to play a role in MCI, according to results from the Mayo Clinic Study of Aging. Participants in the study developed MCI at a rate of about 5.3 percent per year overall. But the rate increased with advanced age. Approximately 3.5 percent of seventy- to seventy-nine-year-olds and about 7.2 percent of eighty- to eighty-nine-year-olds developed the condition each year. Men were nearly twice as likely to develop MCI as were women.

Cognitive capacity among people diagnosed with the disorder seems to devolve more quickly than usual, though not as rapidly as with Alzheimer's, memory specialists say. People who are diagnosed with MCI seem to experience psychiatric symptoms more frequently than those who are cognitively healthy, and anxiety coupled with MCI may be a predictor of Alzheimer's, according to Johns Hopkins memory experts.

Recent research shows that 36 percent of the people with MCI had mood-related depression, 36 percent had motivation-related depression (apathy and withdrawal from social activities, for example), and nearly half (47 percent) showed symptoms of anxiety. By contrast, only 18 percent of cognitively healthy participants had mood-related depression, 13 percent showed symptoms of motivation-related depression, and 25 percent experienced anxiety. Most experts note that they are only beginning to understand MCI, and that its definition and diagnosis are likely to change.

⊑, Essential

"Senior moments" are more likely to occur when you're under stress, tired, sick, or upset. Say, for example, that a coworker asks, at the end of a long workday, for the name of the charming oceanfront bed and breakfast you raved about when you got back from vacation the previous summer. You rack your brain and can't recall it then and there. The following morning the name, address, and proprietor are crystal clear.

Research reported in the May 8, 2007, issue of the journal *Neurology* showed that 83 percent of participants with both MCI and anxiety eventually developed Alzheimer's disease, compared with 41 percent of those with MCI but no anxiety and 6 percent of the cognitively healthy people. In the cognitively healthy group, only depression was linked to the development of AD.

Meanwhile, the American Academy of Neurology has published practice guidelines for diagnosing MCI:

- An individual's report of her own memory problems, preferably confirmed by another person
- Measurable, greater-than-normal memory impairment detected with standard memory assessment tests

- Normal general thinking and reasoning skills
- Ability to perform normal daily activities

Warning Signs of Alzheimer's

The Alzheimer's Association has identified ten warning signs of Alzheimer's disease you should know. To help you better understand those signs, the organization compares symptoms that are cause for concern with those of normal memory loss.

1. **Memory loss.** Forgetting recently learned information, such as names, occurs more frequently. It's normal to forget names or dates occasionally, but it may be cause for concern if you regularly cannot remember important anniversaries or birthdays or have to ask the same questions repeatedly.

2. **Difficulty performing familiar tasks.** You may have trouble planning and finishing everyday tasks or lose track of steps involved preparing a meal, making a phone call, or playing a game. You may not be able to keep track of "notes to self" and other reminders. It's okay if these lapses happen occasionally; making mistakes is a normal part of living.

3. **Problems with language.** People with AD tend to forget simple words or substitute words for those they can't remember. They may search for a telephone, forget what it's called, and ask if you've seen that "talk machine," for instance. It's normal to have trouble finding the right word or forget names of new acquaintances occasionally.

4. **Disorientation to time and place.** People with Alzheimer's disease can become lost in their own neighborhood, forget where they are and how they got there, and not know how to get back home. However, it is normal to forget the day of the week or where you were going.

5. **Poor or questionable judgment.** Someone with AD may wear several layers on a warm day or go out in a T-shirt when there's snow on the ground. Giving away large sums of money to a new charity is also a red flag.

6. **Problems with abstract thinking.** Someone with AD may become befuddled or overwhelmed by complex mental tasks, forgetting what numbers are for and how they should be used. Don't worry if you are finding it more challenging to balance a checkbook.

7. **Routinely misplacing everyday objects and valuable possessions.** A person with Alzheimer's disease may put an iron in the freezer or a wristwatch in the sugar bowl. Temporarily misplacing your keys or wallet is nothing to worry about.

8. **Changes in mood or behavior.** Rapid mood swings—from calm to tears to anger—for no apparent reason is a symptom of AD. It is normal if you occasionally feel sad, moody, or not quite yourself.

9. **Personality changes.** Dementia can change people dramatically. A self-assured, outgoing man may become extremely confused, fearful, or extremely dependent on his wife. However, it is normal for people's personalities to change somewhat with age. You may grow wiser or more impatient.

10. **Loss of initiative.** Apathy and passivity are warning signs. Sitting in front of the TV for hours, sleeping more than usual, or skipping a weekly golf game can signal problems. However, it is normal if you sometimes feel weary of work or social obligations or need to take a mental health day occasionally.

If you are experiencing significant memory problems, see a doctor as soon as possible. Determining what's normal and what isn't is critical to your health and quality of life.

CHAPTER 5

Understanding Alzheimer's Risks

Your age, genes, and family history help determine your risk factors for Alzheimer's disease. But previously unsuspected medical, lifestyle, and environmental factors may also raise your risk. New research indicates that conditions such as diabetes may increase your risk of developing Alzheimer's and even accelerate AD's progression. And while you can't do much about your age, genes, or gender, you may be able to reduce other risks associated with AD.

Debunking Alzheimer's Myths

The first step in understanding your known risks, probable risks, and suspected risks for Alzheimer's is to separate facts from myths—the things "everyone knows"—about AD. Here are ten of the most common:

1. **Myth:** If you live long enough, you're going to get Alzheimer's.

There is no question that aging greatly increases your chances of developing AD. Risk for Alzheimer's doubles every five years after sixty-five. Remember, though, that old age is a risk factor—not a cause of AD.

2. **Myth:** My mother and her aunt had Alzheimer's, so that probably means I'm going to get it too.

In more than 90 percent of cases, heredity is just one risk among many. Genes play a definitive role in a very rare form of AD known as familial early-onset Alzheimer's, which accounts for fewer than 5 percent of Alzheimer diagnoses.

3. **Myth:** A cure for Alzheimer's is right around the corner.

No "magic bullet" that cures, prevents, or even predicts the onset of AD is on the horizon. Scientists expect to find better methods of early detection, diagnosis, and prevention within the next few years. Those may lead to treatments for the disease.

4. **Myth:** There's nothing you can do if you're diagnosed with Alzheimer's disease.

The Food and Drug Administration has approved five drugs that may temporarily relieve some symptoms in some people in the early stages of the disease. A number of treatments can help with sleep disturbance, aggression, depression, and similar problems that afflict people with Alzheimer's, and nondrug therapies can improve quality of life for patients and caregivers.

5. **Myth:** If I'm sure it's Alzheimer's, there's no sense making things worse by getting a medical diagnosis.

You can't be sure it's Alzheimer's or another disease, but you can benefit from treatments designed for people who have been diagnosed with Alzheimer's. It is true that Alzheimer's specialists can only diagnose the disease with certainty when they examine brain tissue unless during an autopsy. Physicians diagnose AD in living patients with 90 percent certainty only after ruling out other brain diseases and possible causes of dementia. Some characteristics of Alzheimer's are observable. Others can only be detected by medical tests administered by a physician or in a lab.

6. **Myth:** There are alternative, natural treatments and cures for AD.

In the absence of a cure or effective treatment for Alzheimer's, hundreds of drugs, procedures, vitamins, and dietary supplements are being tested and retested. Several studies have measured the effectiveness of vitamins E, B, and C and gingko biloba in preventing or treating Alzheimer's disease. Findings so far are mixed and inconclusive, but more investigations are under way.

7. **Myth:** Drinking out of aluminum cans or cooking in aluminum pots and pans can lead to Alzheimer's disease.

This urban legend dates to the 1960s and 1970s, when research showed high aluminum levels in the brain tissue of some people who died with AD. The discovery spurred public concern that exposure to aluminum in pots and pans, beverage cans, antacids, and antiperspirants could cause Alzheimer's. Several scientific studies have examined the link between aluminum and Alzheimer's, and none have found a clear association between aluminum exposure and AD.

Fact

Artificial sweeteners have been accused but never convicted of causing cancer, memory loss, birth defects, brain tumors, multiple sclerosis, Gulf War Syndrome, and brain diseases, including Alzheimer's. No credible scientific evidence so far has proved a connection between aspartame and these diseases.

8. **Myth:** Artificial sweeteners cause memory loss.

The FDA approved aspartame for use in all foods and beverages in 1996 based on what the agency called "a detailed review of a large body of information, including more than 100 toxicological and clinical studies regarding the sweetener's safety." In response to public pressure that arose when one European study suggested aspartame caused cancer in rats, the agency revisited and reconfirmed its original position in 2007. Several studies have confirmed the safety of aspartame for the general public, although it is not considered safe for people who have the rare hereditary disease phenylketonuria (PKU). Products that contain aspartame must carry a PKU warning on the label.

9. **Myth:** Flu shots can put older people at risk for Alzheimer's.

In fact, the opposite may be true. Several scientific studies published in mainstream medical journals link flu shots and other vaccinations to a reduced risk of Alzheimer's disease and overall better health, according to the Alzheimer's Association.

10. **Myth:** Too much worrying or thinking can cause Alzheimer's.

One large, long-term study showed that rumination—thinking carefully and at length about something—actually slowed risk for dementia. The risk was higher among those who fretted less—more so if they were footloose and fancy-free.

Assessing AD Risk

Your chances of developing Alzheimer's are likely affected by your genes, cognitive health, environment, lifestyle, and other factors.

Researchers are seeking ways of defining and measuring these variables to assess your overall risk.

📋 Fact

Your probability of having Alzheimer's is a sum total of a variety of factors, explains neuroscientist Gary Lynch of University of California, Irvine. If, for example, you were born with a particular gene mutation and banged your head on the pavement when you were twelve years old, your chances of having Alzheimer's would be many times greater than someone who had the right genes and wore a helmet biking.

Such varied factors as smoking, head trauma, depression, marital status, and frequency of exercise have all been associated with Alzheimer's. None of these risks predicts your chances of getting AD with any accuracy, but a combination of risks might.

Genetic Risks for Alzheimer's

Teams of scientists around the world are studying the relationship between genes and Alzheimer's, hoping to better understand the pathology of the disease. The discovery of three genetic abnormalities that cause early-onset Alzheimer's and the study of one gene that significantly increases risk for Alzheimer's have adranied scientific understanding of Alzheimer's pathology.

Early-Onset Alzheimer's

Early-onset Alzheimer's (sometimes called younger-onset Alzheimer's) is a rare form of the disease that strikes people between the ages of thirty and sixty, and accounts for fewer than 10 percent of all AD cases. (According to the Alzheimer's Association, some 500,000 people in their thirties, forties, and fifties have Alzheimer's disease or a related dementia.)

A form of early-onset Alzheimer's called early-onset familial Alzheimer's disease (FAD), which accounts for fewer than 5 percent of AD diagnoses overall, is inherited. FAD is caused by mutations in genes on chromosomes 1, 14, or 21, each of which causes excess production of beta-amyloid, a key component of toxic plaques that characterize AD.

Fact

Genes contain the code for the type and order of amino acids needed to build a specific protein. A gene mutation, or defect, can lead to the production of a faulty protein that can cause cell malfunction or disease. Some gene mutations cause defects and diseases. Others raise the risk of developing a disease, but don't assure you'll get it.

FAD is autosomal dominant, which means that if you inherit even one abnormal gene from one parent, you are virtually guaranteed to develop the disease before age sixty-five. Only a few hundred extended families worldwide carry the gene mutations that trigger this rare disease.

EARLY-ONSET ALZHEIMER'S

Early-onset Alzheimer's occasionally strikes people in their early thirties. But most people diagnosed with the rare form of AD are middle-aged, usually in their fifties.

While there is a general impression that early-onset Alzheimer's progresses more rapidly than the far more common late-onset variation in people over age sixty-five, studies show that is not the case, according to Glenn E. Smith, PhD, a neuropsychologist at Mayo Clinic. But symptoms that begin in middle age are unusual, and they may be misdiagnosed—or dismissed—when they initially appear, experts advise. Doctors don't expect to find dementia in a fifty-year-old woman and may suspect her memory problems and confusion are menopause-related, for example. A hard-charging forty-year-old executive's AD symptoms may be diagnosed as stress. Early-onset AD affects the lives of many patients differently, because it develops at a time in life when people with the disease are working and may still have children at home.

"Alzheimer's disease has a tremendous impact at any age," Smith told MayoClinic.com. "But we don't expect to see dementia at a young age, so problems emerging at work or home may be mistakenly ascribed to lack of motivation or diligence, or possible psychiatric problems. People with early-onset Alzheimer's may lose relationships or be fired instead of being identified as medically ill or disabled."

Genes and Late-onset Alzheimer's

Genes play a less definitive role in late-onset Alzheimer's, the far more common form of the disease that affects people ages sixty-five and older.

Scientists have so far identified one risk gene for late-onset Alzheimer's, called Apolipoprotein E4 (ApoE4). It is one of three common variations (or alleles) of the ApoE gene, which codes for a protein that helps carry cholesterol in the bloodstream. Two other common alleles, ApoE2 and ApoE3, are also associated with Alzheimer's, in different ways:

- **ApoE2,** the least common form of the three, is relatively rare. It appears to reduce the risk of Alzheimer's and may delay onset of symptoms in people who get AD.
- **ApoE3,** the most common allele, appears to play a neutral role in Alzheimer's, neither increasing nor decreasing risk.
- **ApoE4,** which is found in approximately 40 percent of people who develop AD, seems to increase risk.

People with an ApoE4 allele inherit an increased risk of developing Alzheimer's, not the disease itself. Some people with one or two ApoE4 alleles never get the disease, and others develop AD without any ApoE4 alleles.

Scientists are still trying to understand how ApoE4 increases your susceptibility to Alzheimer's disease. Some suspect the allele is less involved in whether you get AD than in when you get it. That's because it appears to lower the age at which you develop symptoms and may also speed up progress of the disease. The average age of onset for Alzheimer's symptoms is eighty-four among people with no copies of ApoE4. It's seventy-five in those with one copy (inherited from one parent) and sixty-eight in those with two copies (inherited from both parents).

Fact

Eating a high-fat diet appears to increase Alzheimer's risk. A handful of health practitioners, including Pamela McDonald, an integrative medicine nurse practitioner and author of *The ApoE Gene Diet*, maintain that knowing the combination of ApoE genes you carry can help you modify your diet and make lifestyle changes that can help reduce risk for Alzheimer's and other diseases.

Experts believe there may be as many as a dozen other Alzheimer risk genes in addition to ApoE4. Evidence is building that ApoE4 raises other Alzheimer's risks, including early memory loss, sensitivity to effects of head injuries, and cardiovascular diseases. People with one or two copies of ApoE4 who had a parent with dementia were two to three times more likely to experience memory problems in midlife, according to one large recent study. And people who carry at least one copy of the ApoE4 allele have an increased chance of developing atherosclerosis, the accumulation of fatty deposits and scarlike tissue in the arteries, according to *Genetics Home Reference*, a service of the U.S. National Library of Medicine.

A blood test is available that can identify which ApoE alleles you carry. But because the ApoE4 gene is only a risk factor for AD, the test won't tell you with any certainty whether you will develop the disease.

Most Alzheimer's experts discourage genetic testing for ApoE4. But that thinking may change as science learns more about genetic and lifestyle risks for Alzheimer's, according to Dr. Murali Doraiswamy and Lisa Gwyther, authors of *The Alzheimer's Action Plan*. They urge anyone who is considering the ApoE4 screen to consider the following issues:

- Most insurance plans won't cover ApoE testing.
- One in four people—approximately 25 percent of the U.S. population—carry one copy of the ApoE4 gene and will test positive.
- Half of all people with Alzheimer's do not test positive. The fact that you don't carry the gene doesn't mean you won't develop AD.
- At least 20 percent of people with ApoE4 do not develop Alzheimer's.
- Whether or when someone with ApoE4 develops AD depends on many factors, including other diseases and lifestyle risks.
- Inheriting one copy of the ApoE4 gene puts you at approximately the same risk as having a parent with Alzheimer's.

As Doraiswamy and Gwyther see it, the ApoE4 is a less-than-perfect predictor whose results may cause people to become anxious or despondent. But ApoE4 testing in the proper context—as part of a research study that provides comprehensive testing and genetic counseling, for example—may provide useful information to ApoE4 carriers, encouraging them to protect themselves against high cholesterol.

Other Established Risks for Alzheimer's

While it appears that there is no single cause for AD, certain factors are known to increase risk for the disease.

Age

The vast majority of people with Alzheimer's are sixty-five or older. One in eight people over sixty-five and nearly half of those who live past eighty-five suffer from Alzheimer's or a related dementia, according to the American Academy of Neurology.

ESTIMATED RISK OF DEVELOPING ALZHEIMER'S

Age	Risk
61–70	1%
71–80	2.3%
81–90	18.1%
90+	29.7%

Gender

One in six women and one in ten men who live to age fifty-five will develop Alzheimer's disease in their remaining lifetimes. Older women aren't really at greater risk than men their age for Alzheimer's, experts say. But because women tend to live longer, more of them develop the disease.

Essential

Remember, most octogenarians do not develop dementia. If they did, people who have played vital roles in international arenas while they were in their eighties—Nelson Mandela, former presidents George H.W. Bush and Jimmy Carter, Pope Benedict XVI, and a slew of Supreme Court justices—would be absent from the world stage.

Any other gender difference is probably influenced by estrogen, the primary female hormone, which appears to offer some protection against memory loss and cognitive decline. Estrogen levels drop after menopause, and that could explain the higher risk in older women than in men. But studies of whether and how much the decline in natural estrogen levels affects older women's mental functions have been inconclusive.

Down Syndrome

Approximately one in four people with Down syndrome who are ages thirty-five or older develop symptoms of Alzheimer's disease. The percentage increases with age. The incidence of Alzheimer's among people with Down syndrome is estimated to be three to five times greater than it is among the general population.

Probable Risks for Alzheimer's

Increasing evidence has linked brain injury, inflammation, and emotional conditions with memory loss and dementia.

Head Injury

Suffering a head injury in early adulthood appears to increase Alzheimer's risk later in life, according to the National Institute of Neurological Disorders and Stroke. The more severe the head injury, the greater the risk. Some experts suspect that head injuries interact with other factors to trigger AD, and that traumatic brain injuries (TBIs) may speed up onset of symptoms in people who are already at risk.

Fact

TBIs occur more frequently in the United States than do breast cancer or AIDS, according to the Centers for Disease Control and Prevention (CDC), which estimates that one out of every fifty Americans are currently living with disabilities from TBI.

Inflammation

Brain tissue inflammation is commonly observed in people diagnosed with AD. Scientists aren't sure whether inflammation—the body's response to infection, irritation, or other injury—is a cause or effect of degenerative brain disease. AD researchers have studied and are actively investigating the role that nonsteroidal anti-inflammatory drugs (NSAIDs) such as naproxen (Aleve) might play in preventing or slowing the progression of the disease.

UNDERSTANDING CAUSE AND RISK

If you read or listen to science and health news, you might think that memory loss, head injury, and advanced age cause Alzheimer's disease, and that drinking coffee, doing crossword puzzles, and getting a college degree prevent it. It's good to know how and why that isn't so. Many people confuse cause with risk (or correlation). For the record:

- A cause makes something happen; it results in a predictable reaction. There is a direct line between cause and effect. (HIV causes AIDS. Heart failure causes death.)
- A risk correlates (or is associated) with an event or disease. It may increase the likelihood of something occurring, but it doesn't guarantee it will.

Here are some examples: There is no question that advanced age is closely associated with Alzheimer's disease. The older you get, the greater your risk for AD. But old age doesn't cause Alzheimer's; if it did, everyone over age sixty-five would have the disease. Similarly, having a college education has been associated with a decreased risk for Alzheimer's (and there are many possible explanations for this). But having a degree doesn't prevent Alzheimer's.

Pay close attention to news reports about the supposed causes of a disease like Alzheimer's. The headlines may suggest that diabetes causes Alzheimer's. But the stories themselves will likely use qualifiers—"may be linked," "might increase," "could increase the risk"—to distinguish cause from correlation or risk.

Lifestyle Risks

According to the Centers for Disease Control and Prevention (CDC), the average seventy-five-year-old has three chronic medical conditions and takes five prescription medicines. Most Americans over age sixty-five suffer from hypertension, nearly one in five have diabetes, and two out of three are overweight. Obese people are twice as likely to suffer from dementia, and people with diabetes are at far greater risk for developing Alzheimer's disease, federal health officials say. All of this matters if you're concerned about brain health, because the conditions and diseases that destroy your body damage your brain as well.

 Alert

Watch out for belly fat, even if you're not obese or overweight. People whose bellies bulge when they're in their forties are more likely to develop Alzheimer's and other forms of dementia thirty years later, researchers reported in the journal *Neurology*.

The following conditions or lifestyle factors may contribute to the likelihood that someone may develop Alzheimer's disease:

- **Diabetes.** A debilitating and incurable condition in which the body has trouble breaking down sugars, diabetes is the sixth leading cause of death in the United States. It is known to raise the risk of heart disease and kidney failure. Diabetes also increases the risk of Alzheimer's disease and vascular dementia, according to the American Diabetes Association. The risk is stronger when diabetes occurs at midlife than in late life.
- **Atherosclerosis.** Atherosclerosis is the buildup of plaque—deposits of fatty substances, cholesterol, and other matter—in the inner lining of an artery. Atherosclerosis is a

significant risk factor for vascular dementia, because it interferes with the delivery of blood to the brain and can lead to stroke. Studies have also found a possible link between atherosclerosis and AD.

- **Cholesterol.** High levels of low-density lipoprotein (LDL), the so-called "bad" form of cholesterol, appear to significantly increase a person's risk of developing vascular dementia. Some research has also linked high cholesterol to a significantly increased risk for AD.

- **Metabolic syndrome.** This describes a group of heart disease risk factors—abdominal obesity, elevated blood pressure, high triglycerides, elevated blood sugar, and low HDL ("good") cholesterol—that increase risk for developing diabetes, hypertension, and stroke. All three of these conditions increase the risk of developing dementia, including Alzheimer's disease.

- **Homocysteine.** High levels of this amino acid in the blood are tied to higher risk of coronary heart disease, stroke, and vascular disease and may also elevate risk for Alzheimer's.

- **Smoking.** Several studies show that smoking cigarettes significantly raises the risk of mental decline and dementia. That may be because people who smoke have a higher risk of atherosclerosis and other types of vascular disease, which can cause increased dementia risk.

- **Alcohol use.** Alcoholics are at higher risk for dementia. But people who drink moderately—no more than two drinks daily for men and no more than one for women—seem to be better protected from dementia than are alcohol abusers and abstainers, according to current research. What's more, drinking moderate amounts of red wine may offer some protection from Alzheimer's disease, researchers reported in the *Journal of Biological Chemistry* in November 2008. Naturally occurring compounds in red wine called *polyphenols* appear to block formation of the beta-amyloid proteins that build toxic plaques in the brains of people with AD.

Psychological Risks: Depression and Stress

People who are prone to distress, depression, and loneliness appear to be at greater risk of Alzheimer's.

Depression

Estimates of the number of people diagnosed with AD who suffer significant depression range from 40 to 70 percent, and people who treat Alzheimer's patients have long assumed that being depressed is a symptom or response to the disease.

But some experts believe depression may be a cause, not an effect, of Alzheimer's disease. That was the conclusion of a large thirteen-year study at Rush University Medical Center, in which 40 percent of participants were diagnosed with both AD and depression.

Alert

The fact that depression and anxiety are risk factors for memory loss may actually be good news. Strategies that reduce anxiety and depression can improve mental health and well-being, and that may help prevent memory loss.

Starting in the early 1990s, Rush researchers tracked the cognitive health of 917 older Catholic priests, nuns, and brothers in the Religious Orders Study at Rush University. None of the participants had Alzheimer's or another dementia at the outset of the study, and 53.6 percent of participants reported no symptoms of depression. Among the group, 23.9 percent reported one symptom of depression, 9.7 percent reported two, and the rest reported three or more, according to the study's lead investigator, Robert S. Wilson.

Study volunteers underwent yearly clinical evaluations that included cognitive testing and assessment of depressive symptoms. During the study period, 190 participants developed

Alzheimer's. Those who did showed no increase in depressive symptoms in the years leading up to diagnosis, when they were experiencing early signs of cognitive decline. Nor was there a general increase in their depression after their diagnoses, researchers reported.

However, those who had symptoms of depression at the beginning of the study were more likely to develop AD. If Alzheimer's disease caused depression, depressive symptoms would be apparent in the years before and after diagnosis—which usually coincides with the onset of cognitive decline, according to Wilson. That didn't happen. But the correlation between depression at the start of the study and in those with AD seems to support Wilson's contention that depression may be a risk factor for Alzheimer's.

DEPRESSION AND ALZHEIMER'S DISEASE

Depression and Alzheimer's disease often go hand in hand. Depression can mask Alzheimer's, it may be mistaken Alzheimer's, and it may exacerbate the disease. Depression sometimes precedes the onset of AD symptoms or develops as those symptoms occur.

Depression doesn't "look" the same in people with Alzheimer's as it does in other people, dementia experts warn. It is sometimes less severe. Depressive bouts may not last as long or recur as often as they do in other people.

People with cognitive problems may not be able to express their feelings of sadness, hopelessness, guilt, and other emotions we associate with depression. They may be less likely to talk openly about wanting to kill themselves, and they are less likely to attempt suicide than are depressed individuals without dementia, according to Alzheimer's Association experts, who point out that "depressive symptoms in Alzheimer's may come and go, in contrast to memory and thinking problems that worsen steadily over time."

Assessing Depression

These questions, drawn from what's known as the geriatric depression scale, can help you determine if you or another older person is depressed. This assessment is used by the American Geriatrics Society. First, answer these questions:

1. Are you basically satisfied with your life?
2. Have you dropped many of your activities and interests?
3. Do you feel that your life is empty?
4. Do you often get bored?
5. Are you in good spirits most of the time?
6. Are you afraid that something bad is going to happen to you?
7. Do you feel happy most of the time?
8. Do you often feel helpless?
9. Do you prefer to stay at home, rather than going out and doing new things?
10. Do you feel you have more problems with memory than most?
11. Do you think it is wonderful to be alive now?
12. Do you feel pretty worthless the way you are now?
13. Do you feel full of energy?
14. Do you feel that your situation is hopeless?
15. Do you think that most people are better off than you are?

Tally your points according to the key.
1. Yes: 0 points.   No: 1 point.
2. Yes: 1 point.   No: 0 points
3. Yes: 1 point.   No: 0 points.
4. Yes: 1 point.   No: 0 points.
5. Yes: 0 points.   No: 1 point.
6. Yes: 1 point   No: 0 points.
7. Yes: 0 points.   No: 1 point.

8. Yes: 1 point   No: 0 points.
9. Yes: 1 point.   No: 0 points.
10. Yes: 1 point.   No: 0 points.
11. Yes: 0 points.   No: 1 point.
12. Yes: 1 point.   No: 0 points.
13. Yes: 0 points.   No: 1 point.
14. Yes: 1 point.   No: 0 points.
15. Yes: 1 point.   No: 0 points.

If your score is five or higher, you may have symptoms of depression. Speak to a trusted counselor or clinician about this soon.

Stress

Excess levels of the stress hormone cortisol can interfere with brain function, particularly memory. In response to a threat, your adrenal glands release adrenalin. If the threat is serious—or lasts more than a couple of minutes—the adrenals release cortisol.

Research conducted as part of the ongoing Baltimore Memory Study has linked high levels of cortisol with a decline in cognitive performance among older people.

Cortisol remains in the brain longer than adrenalin; it irritates brain cells and interferes with the function of neurotransmitters, the chemicals that enable your brain cells to communicate. Too much cortisol can damage your hippocampus, the part of the brain central to learning and memory. That can make it difficult to think clearly or retrieve long-term memories during a crisis.

Environmental Risks for Alzheimer's

Your racial or ethnic background, how long you go to school, and the work you do all influence your risk for dementia.

Education

People with fewer years of education appear to be at greater risk for AD and other dementias. No one is quite sure why, but a slew of studies show that someone who did not complete high school is more likely to develop dementia than is someone who graduated from college. Some experts say that learning itself stimulates brain cell growth. They speculate that years spent in college or graduate school may help build up individual cognitive reserve, which may help protect against Alzheimer's or keep it at bay longer.

Highly educated people are also likely to have more mentally stimulating jobs, better overall physical health, and more disposable income to spend on exercise, travel and other activities that are believed to enhance brain health.

In addition, it may be difficult to detect Alzheimer's disease in people with sixteen or more years of education, who can often compensate for—or hide—early symptoms of memory loss, clinicians say. Better-educated people tend to be diagnosed with dementia later in the course of the disease, once their symptoms become impossible to ignore. They tend to decline quickly following diagnoses made relatively late in the course of the disease.

Better educated people also score higher on a standard screening test for cognitive function, the mini-mental state examination (MMSE), according to a large study reported in the July 2008 *Archives of Neurology*. Researchers and Texas Tech University and Mayo Clinic Medical School recommended that older patients who score less than a 27 out of 30 on the MMSE should receive further evaluations if they have a college or graduate education. This differs from the standard MMSE recommendations, which set a score of 24 or below as the threshold for prompting further evaluations.

THE SCHOOL SISTERS OF NOTRE DAME

Some of the earliest evidence that keeping your brain active and engaged may guard against dementia emerged not in a test lab or academic research center, but from a community of Catholic religious women, the School Sisters of Notre Dame in Mankato, Minnesota. Epidemiologist David Snowdon happened upon the evidence while studying healthy aging among the sisters during the mid-1980s. As he gathered information on the sisters' life histories and lifelong habits, his research confirmed what earlier studies had suggested: that having a college education and active intellectual life appear to protect some people against the ravages of AD. While all the aging sisters had some intellectual decline, Snowdon found that those who had gone to college and taught most of their lives declined less than did sisters who did service jobs.

But Snowdon was able to go further than other epidemiologists in linking intellectual activity in younger adulthood to brain health in old age thanks to an archive at the convent. The sisters in Mankato community had all written autobiographies when they entered the convent as young women, in their twenties.

Working with linguistics experts, Snowdon compared autobiographies with their cognitive health in late life and found a remarkable correlation between the sophistication of thought and optimism expressed and cognitive health later in life. The nuns who had written the most verbally expressive, upbeat essays showed fewer signs of intellectual decline half a century later.

However, this study raises a chicken-and-egg question that continues to dominate epidemiological research about intellectual activity and dementia: Were the sisters who wrote the lower-scoring essays hobbled even in young adulthood by early signs of cognitive decline? Or were those who wrote richer, more complex youthful biographies protected from developing symptoms of dementia?

Class, Race, and Ethnicity

Low education levels are closely linked with poverty, poor diet, and malnutrition; high levels of hypertension, cardiovascular disease, and diabetes; and restricted access to health and medical care. People who struggle to feed, house, and support their families often don't have the money, time, or exposure to health education. African Americans and Latinos who are under-educated, impoverished, and in poor health appear to be at extremely high risk for dementia.

Fact

Latinos with diabetes, high blood pressure, or heart disease are less likely to receive services to help monitor and control those conditions, according to a report by the Alzheimer's Association. Barriers to the health care system can delay identification and diagnosis of dementia, leading to higher levels of impairment among people with the disease.

As a group, African Americans are more likely to suffer heart disease and stroke than is the rest of the American population. They also appear to be at increased risk for diabetes, high blood pressure, high cholesterol, and cardiovascular complications. Alzheimer's Association researchers point out, however, that these worrisome statistics describe African Americans of all educational levels and socioeconomic backgrounds, and that educated middle-class and upper-middle-class African Americans seem to face much the same risks for Alzheimer's and dementia as do Caucasians.

A vast, enormously diverse population that includes people of all races and from twenty-five countries of origin, Latinos are not genetically predisposed to Alzheimer's. However, they do face many risk factors for AD.

A disproportionate number of Hispanic Americans are sixty-five and older, an age that categorically puts them at greater risk for

Alzheimer's disease. Low-income, less educated Hispanic Americans also appear to be at elevated risk for vascular disease, including diabetes, which has been linked to dementia

STATISTICS OF CAREGIVERS

African-American and Hispanic caregivers were more likely than caregivers of other races to think Alzheimer's is a normal part of aging, according to a 2007 survey conducted by the Alzheimer's Foundation of America. Thirty-seven percent of African-American, 33 percent of Latino, and 23 percent of Caucasian caregivers said they considered AD part and parcel of old age. Seventy percent of African-American and 67 percent of Hispanic caregivers were more likely to dismiss the symptoms of Alzheimer's as old age, compared with 53 percent of caregivers of other races.

In addition, 67 percent of African-American and 63 percent of Hispanic caregivers were also more likely to say they didn't know enough about Alzheimer's to recognize its symptoms, compared with 49 percent of caregivers of other races. However, 33 percent of African-American and 26 percent of Hispanic caregivers thought they were at higher risk for Alzheimer's than did caregivers of other races, only 12 percent of whom considered themselves at risk.

Public health surveys show that Hispanics are less likely than other Americans to see doctors, in part because of financial and language barriers. They more often mistake dementia symptoms for normal aging, delaying diagnosis and inadvertently exacerbating the effects of the disease.

CHAPTER 6

Can Alzheimer's Be Prevented?

A merican baby boomers, determined to beat back Alzheimer's, are driving a multi-billion-dollar cottage industry for brain health. The market for neuro software (or brain fitness software) was $225 million in 2007, and it has been growing by 50 percent each year, according to Alvaro Fernandez, cofounder and chief executive officer of SharpBrains, a brain fitness and consulting company. However, scientists warn that no pill, tool, or game is a proven deterrent to dementia. Most urge people who are concerned about brain health to stay mentally sharp, physically fit, and socially engaged.

Move Your Body, Maintain Your Brain

If you exercise to reduce your risk of heart attack, stroke, and diabetes, you may also be protecting yourself against Alzheimer's and other dementias. Regular exercisers have lower rates of cardiovascular disease, type 2 diabetes, high blood pressure, and obesity—all conditions that appear to influence risk for AD.

Scientists and clinicians have known for some time that vigorous physical activity improves brain function because it increases blood flow to the brain. More recently, they have learned that exercise stimulates brain cell activity, spurring the growth of dense, interconnected webs that make the brain run faster and more efficiently, according to Harvard psychiatrist John J. Ratey, MD, author of *Spark: The Revolutionary New Science of Exercise and the Brain*.

"All these structural changes improve your brain's ability to learn and remember, execute higher thought processes, and manage your emotions," says Dr. Ratey. "The more robust the connections, the better prepared your brain will be to handle any damage it might experience."

Exercise and Dementia

Exercise appears to help prevent some of the brain atrophy (shrinkage) that characterizes AD. Early-stage Alzheimer's patients who were more physically fit had larger brains than did those who were less physically fit, scientists announced in summer 2008. Decreasing brain volume has been tied to poorer cognitive performance. Using reams of data they gathered from the Religious Orders Study and the Rush Memory and Aging Project, researchers have identified environmental and lifestyle factors that seem to influence cognitive reserve:

❑ Habitual conscientiousness—always being conscientious, not only at certain times or in regard to certain matters
❑ Years of education
❑ Maintaining strong social networks
❑ Lifelong participation in mentally stimulating activities

Scientists' best guess about the benefits of these characteristics is that each and every one stimulates mental activity, which may enhance brain cell growth and build up cognitive reserve. Some compare cognitive reserve to having extra cash in your bank account for a rainy day. If catastrophe strikes and you have some extra money, you'll be able to live more comfortably for longer than you would if you had no savings. Similarly, cognitive reserve may allow you to ward off or compensate for the earliest signs of dementia.

Researchers note, too, that the characteristics themselves may be interrelated. Conscientious people often do well enough in grammar and high school that they go to college, where many people form friendships and pursue extracurricular interests and activities. College-educated people tend to have more leisure time and money for stimulating pursuits like theater- and concert-going or extended travel.

Factors that work against healthy brain aging and seem to reduce brain reserve include the following:

❑ Being prone to distress
❑ Loneliness
❑ Depression

Evidence is building that ties depression to cognitive decline. Depression has a corrosive effect on the hippocampus, the brain's center of learning and memory, which is particularly vulnerable to age-related nerve cell loss, says Dr. Ratey. Anxiety, which produces stress, can also wreak havoc in the hippocampus.

Essential

Physical activities that involve mental engagement, such as plotting a route, observing traffic signals, and making choices, can add value to your brain health workout—particularly if you do these activities with a companion, according to the Alzheimer's Association.

No one is yet certain why exercise may protect against Alzheimer's, but some experts suspect it may slow the buildup of plaque that accumulates in brains of people with AD. Exercise also helps prevent inflammation, which is frequently observed in brains of Alzheimer's patients. In addition, exercise appears to help beat the blues.

What Exercise Works Best

Aerobic exercise is elemental to physical fitness. Just thirty minutes a day of moderately intense physical exercise—running, biking, or swimming—can improve your memory, sharpen your thinking, and help you handle multitasking, experts on healthy aging say.

Several studies show that walking regularly can benefit your brain. Walking increases blood circulation and the amounts of oxygen and glucose that reach your brain, science educators at the Franklin Institute point out. When you walk, you effectively oxygenate your brain. Senior citizens who walk regularly show significant improvement in their memory skills, learning ability, concentration, and abstract reasoning.

Question

Can playing golf help save your brain?
Golf isn't a sport known for its aerobic benefits. But playing eighteen holes without a cart involves physical exercise (walking as well as swinging), mental stimulation (strategizing and keeping score), and social contact.

Evidence continues to build that strength training enhances the benefits of aerobic exercise and provides perks of its own. The stronger your muscles, the longer you will be able to get up from a chair by yourself, lift your grandchildren, and walk through a park. Keeping your muscles in shape also helps prevent falls. Strength training helps preserve bones as well.

Flexibility exercises, including stretching routines and yoga, which help your body stay limber, can reduce stress and help improve sleep, mood, and overall health. Yoga, tai chi, and balance exercises can also help prevent a serious threat to older people's physical and mental health: falls.

A 1999 Duke University study called SMILE (Standard Medical Intervention and Long-Term Exercise) showed that regular aerobic exercise was as effective at diminishing depression as was Zoloft, a frequently prescribed antidepressant. Exercise rallies brain chemicals that are proven mood lifters and increases brain production of dopamine, a neurotransmitter that stimulates the brain's motivation and reward center.

Avoid Falls

Falls are not inevitable as you age. But they tend to occur most often among older adults with limited mobility, chronic health problems, and poor vision.

Falls are the most frequent cause of hip, spine, limb, and other skeletal fractures in elderly people. Falls also cause tens of thousands of traumatic brain injuries (TBIs) in Americans sixty-five and older each year, according to the Centers for Disease Control and Prevention (CDC). In 2005, nearly 16,000 older adults died from falls, 1.8 million older adults were treated in emergency departments for injuries related to falls, and 433,000 of these patients were hospitalized.

Fact

TBIs caused by a bump or blow to the head during an accident in which a bone is fractured and treated may be missed or misdiagnosed, leading to long-term cognitive, emotional, or functional impairments, according to the CDC.

Older people who fall and aren't injured may become anxious about losing their balance. Some shy away from physical and social activities. Decreased activity impedes mobility, fitness, and balance—and increases the risk of another fall.

AT RUSH UNIVERSITY RELIGIOUS ORDERS STUDY

A group of Roman Catholic nuns, priests, and brothers signed on in 1994 for an unusual mission: helping Alzheimer's researchers study and discover changes in the aging brain. Since then, more than 1,000 religious men and women have participated in the Rush Religious Orders Study, which has provided reams of clinical and pathological data in groundbreaking investigations of possible Alzheimer's risks such as depression and social isolation. Evidence from the Rush Religious Orders Study formed the basis of recent evidence showing that depression may be a risk factor for Alzheimer's, rather than a symptom of the disease.

Centered at the Rush University Medical Center in Chicago and funded through 2011 by the National Institute on Aging, the study has followed most of its subjects for thirteen years. All participants have normal cognitive function at the outset and undergo comprehensive medical, neurological, psychological, and cognitive testing each year. All volunteers donate their brains after death.

Members of religious orders are willing—and welcome—to study volunteers. Their backgrounds and lifestyles tend to be similar, which makes it easier for researchers to identify or rule out important risk factors. Few nuns, priests, and brothers smoke or drink, almost none have children, and they engage in similar work and leisure activities. That means researchers have fewer "variables" to adjust for in studying members of religious orders than they do with other adult groups.

Many members of Catholic religious orders are motivated volunteers. Some are educators who respect the advancement of knowledge; many are altruists who are interested in improving the lives of others. They also tend to live together in communities, making recruitment, retention, and yearly follow-up far less challenging than it is with the general population.

It's important to note that the Religious Orders Study and most studies of lifestyle factors, risks, and prevention are large epidemiological studies—studies based on population—that look at certain behaviors and use statistical methods to relate those behaviors to health outcomes. These studies can show an association or correlation between a factor (exercise) and an outcome (lower rate of dementia). But they don't demonstrate or prove cause and effect. The gold standard for showing scientific evidence of cause and effect is a clinical trial. (See Chapter 13 for more about clinical trials.)

Always Connect

AD experts have known for some time that single people are at higher risk for cognitive decline than are people who live with a partner or spouse. But the reason you are single may further affect AD risk.

Fact

Just reading a daily newspaper could help ward off dementia and Alzheimer's disease. Cognitively active seniors who read, play cards or board games, and do home repairs or engage in other stimulating mental activities were 2.6 times less likely to develop dementia and Alzheimer's than were cognitively inactive people, according to researchers at the Rush University Medical Center in Chicago.

Unmarried people are at twice the risk of developing Alzheimer's as their married counterparts, according to a twenty-one-year Swedish research study of more than 1,400 people. Study subjects who lived with a partner in midlife were less likely to be cognitively impaired than all the others, including those who were widowed, single, divorced, or separated. Those who were living with a partner at midlife also had a 50 percent lower risk of developing dementia in late life than did those who lived alone. This was true even after the researchers adjusted their figures to take into account factors such as weight, physical activity, and education.

By contrast, people who stayed single their whole lives had a doubled risk of dementia. Those who were divorced from midlife onward were at triple the normal risk for dementia. Subjects who were widowed before midlife and remained single had more than a six-fold risk of developing Alzheimer's than did their married counterparts.

Question

Are some leisure activities more protective than others?
A study of 800 men and women ages seventy-five and older showed that those who were physically, socially, and mentally active had a lower risk for developing dementia than did the sedentary seniors in the group. Those who combined different activities—walking and talking with a friend, for example—did even better.

Marriage provides social and intellectual stimulation, both of which appear to protect cognitive health, study author Krister Hakansson of the Karolinska Institutet in Stockholm told fellow researchers at the International Conference on Alzheimer's Disease (ICAD 2008) in Chicago. "Living in a couple relationship is normally one of the most intense forms of social and intellectual stimulation. It means that you are confronted with other ideas, perspectives, and needs. You have to compromise, make decisions, and solve problems together with someone else, which is more complicated and challenging. It is probably easier to get stuck in your own habits and routines if you live by yourself."

The Importance of Being Social

Put away your remote and make some plans. Lonely people may be twice as likely to develop dementia linked to Alzheimer's disease in late life as those who are not lonely. People with strong networks of friends and family are less vulnerable to memory loss and dementia, aging experts say. Those with the highest social integration had the slowest rate of memory decline in recent studies.

Essential

You probably don't need experts to tell you that surrounding yourself with supportive family, friends, and coworkers makes you feel better. You've formed social networks throughout adult life—at work, in the neighborhood, or in your community. Building a social network after retirement takes a little more effort, but it's essential to your health.

Social integration, which was measured on the basis of marital status, volunteer activities, and contact with parents, children, and neighbors, had a protective effect on older adults' cognitive health regardless of age, gender, race, and health status, according to a Harvard School of Public Health study funded by the National Institute on Aging. Memory loss among the most socially integrated was less than half what it was among the least integrated.

Diet

Following a heart-friendly, brain-healthy diet low in fat and cholesterol reduces your risk of heart disease and diabetes and encourages the flow of healthy blood to your brain. Managing body weight is crucial to maintaining physical and cognitive health, say national health officials. People who are obese in their forties are 74 percent more likely to develop dementia compared to those of normal weight, according to the National Institutes of Health.

Brain Food

Eating protective foods thought to reduce the risk of heart disease and stroke may also protect brain cells, nutrition experts at the Alzheimer's Association say. A brain-healthy diet is rich in foods containing vitamins B12, C, E, and folate, as well as antioxidants and omega-3 fatty acids. Among foods you may want to try are the following:

- **Dark-skinned vegetables and fruits.** Kale, spinach, broccoli, beets, onions, and eggplant generally have the highest levels of naturally occurring antioxidants. Prunes, raisins, blueberries, blackberries, strawberries, raspberries, plums, oranges, red grapes, and cherries have high antioxidant levels as well.
- **Cold-water fish.** Halibut, mackerel, salmon, trout, and tuna are good sources of beneficial omega-3 fatty acids, which may reduce age-related cognitive decline.
- **Certain kinds of nuts.** Almonds, pecans, and walnuts are a good source of vitamin E, which is an antioxidant.

ALZHEIMER'S AND THE MEDITERRANEAN DIET

A diet laden with fish, olive oil, veggies, and other staples of Mediterranean-style cuisine may help fend off mild cognitive impairment (MCI), as well as Alzheimer's disease. (See Chapter 4 for more information about MCI.) Indeed, such a diet may actually reduce the likelihood that MCI would decline into full-fledged Alzheimer's, according to research reported by Columbia University Medical Center in *Archives of Neurology* in 2009. The study was yet another heaping endorsement of the Mediterranean diet, which also protects against cholesterol, hypertension, diabetes, and other cardiovascular risks, as a way to brain health.

The research team examined, interviewed, and screened 1,393 individuals with healthy brains and 482 patients with mild cognitive impairment over an average of four and a half years. During that time, 275 of the 1,393 study participants who did not have MCI at the outset developed the condition. Subjects who adhered most strictly to a Mediterranean diet—rich in vegetables, legumes, and fish, and low in fat, meat, and dairy—had a 28 percent lower risk of developing mild cognitive impairment than did the one-third of participants who ate the fewest foods related to the Mediterranean diet. The middle one-third had a 17 percent lower risk of developing mild cognitive impairment than did those who ate the fewest Mediterranean foods.

Of the 482 study participants who had mild cognitive impairment at the beginning of the study, 106 developed Alzheimer's disease roughly four years later. The one-third of participants who followed the Mediterranean diet most closely had a 48 percent less risk of developing Alzheimer's than did the one-third with the lowest diet scores.

Vitamins and Dietary Supplements

Rigorous studies of vitamin supplements that showed some promise of preventing or delaying dementia have produced decidedly mixed results. No vitamin, dietary supplements, or complementary treatment can prevent, reverse, or cure symptoms of Alzheimer's disease. Alternative treatments for Alzheimer's symptoms—gingko biloba, folate, vitamin B, and vitamin E—have yet to prove effective and safe in large, rigorous scientific studies. Manufacturers of those supplements continue to market them as antidotes to Alzheimer's, but be aware that they may not have any scientific evidence to back up their claims. Unlike prescription and over-the-counter drugs, the herbal remedies, vitamins, and other dietary supplements are not required to prove their effectiveness or safety before they are marketed and sold in the United States.

Vitamin E

Antioxidants such as vitamins E and C can neutralize free radicals that circulate in your bloodstream, and they may protect nerve cells in the brain. Many theorize that antioxidants may protect against dementia, and in fact one large federally funded study during the 1990s showed that taking large doses of vitamin E slightly delayed loss of cognitive ability in Alzheimer's patients.

Alert

> Though vitamin E may have other health benefits, few doctors recommend the supplements as a treatment for dementia, and Alzheimer's experts warn against taking the supplement unless you are under a physician's supervision. High doses of vitamin E can interact with other medications and may also prevent blood clotting in older adults.

However, scientific studies since that time haven't really indicated that vitamins E or C provide brain protection, even at high doses. A large five-year study published in the Journal of the American Geriatrics Society in February 2008 showed no reduced risk for dementia or AD among older adults who use over-the-counter vitamin E or C supplements. That was true even among subjects who took both vitamins, hoping the combination might offer greater protection, and among older adults who took E at higher than normally recommended doses.

Ginkgo Biloba

A staple of traditional Chinese medicine for centuries, gingko biloba is a plant extract thought to have both antioxidant and anti-inflammatory effects. It is used in Europe to treat cognitive symptoms of neurological disorders, and preliminary studies in the United States indicated that it might enhance brain health.

But the Gingko Evaluation of Memory (GEM) study, the largest, longest independent clinical trial of ginkgo biloba's effectiveness in preventing memory loss, surprised and disappointed those who had high hopes for the supplements' effectiveness and safety.

Researchers from five academic medical centers followed 3,069 volunteers ages seventy-five and older for approximately six years, and found that gingko supplements neither prevented nor delayed dementia or Alzheimer's disease. The researchers reported in the *Journal of the American Medical Association* (JAMA) in 2008 that most participants were cognitively healthy at the outset of the trial, though some had mild cognitive impairment, and that half took two doses of 120 milligrams of ginkgo biloba extract daily and half were given placebo pills. The study was double-blind, meaning that neither the participants nor the study staff knew who was receiving gingko supplements and who was taking a placebo.

Fact

Americans spent about $107 million on ginkgo biloba supplements in the United States in 2007, according to *Consumer Reports*. A year's supply of the supplement can cost about $200 per person.

During the course of the study, 523 participants were diagnosed with dementia. Of those, 246, or 16.1 percent, were taking placebos; 277, or 17.9 percent, were taking ginkgo biloba.

Gingko is generally well tolerated, which means that most people can take it without experiencing side effects. It has, however, been associated with slight increases in strokes and ministrokes, and with irregular bleeding. Ginkgo inhibits the action of platelets in the blood and can interfere with blood coagulation, or clotting, according to federal health officials, who warn against taking ginkgo if you are taking the blood thinner warfarin (Coumadin) or antiplatelet drugs such as clopidogrel (Plavix). Ginkgo may lower blood sugar, so people taking drugs for diabetes should avoid gingko as well.

In the GEM study, researchers reported no difference in heart attack or ischemic strokes between the ginkgo and placebo-treated patients. There were more hemorrhagic (bleeding) strokes among the ginkgo group, though the number of cases was not significant, they noted. According to the study's authors, the possible adverse effects of gingko bolstered the case against recommending the supplement.

Coenzyme Q10

Coenzyme Q10 (CoQ10), or ubiquinone, is an antioxidant that occurs naturally in the body and is needed for normal cell reactions. CoQ10 levels, which decrease with age, appear to be low in people with certain chronic diseases.

Fact

An estimated 73 percent of Americans ages sixty-five and older are overweight, according to the Centers for Disease Control and Prevention. Simply being overweight can double your chances of developing dementia.

You can increase levels of CoQ10 in your body by taking CoQ10 supplements, medical experts say, but it is not clear that replacing low CoQ10 is beneficial or that it will counteract disease. CoQ10 has been used, recommended, or studied for numerous conditions, but it remains controversial as a treatment in many areas.

Some preliminary evidence suggests that CoQ10 supplements may slow some symptoms of dementia in people with Alzheimer's.

Omega-3

Studies of the omega-3 fatty acid docosahexaenoic acid (DHA), which is found in fatty fish and fish oil, suggest it shows some promise as a brain booster. The most abundant fatty acid in your brain, DHA is crucial to normal vision and brain function. It is also a natural anti-inflammatory and antioxidant agent. Clinical trials are investigating indications that people with high levels of DHA in their bloodstreams may be at reduced risk for Alzheimer's and that omega-3 fatty acid supplements may slow decline in very early AD.

Folate and B Vitamins

Claims that large doses of B vitamins might minimize brain deterioration in people with AD were undercut in 2008, when clinical trials of high-dose supplements of folate and vitamins B6 and B12 showed no effect on the symptoms of people with mild and moderate Alzheimer's.

Question

Do any supplements show promise?
Several dietary supplements that may help stave off or slow cognitive decline are under investigation. Researchers are testing the combined effects of antioxidants (vitamin E, vitamin C, alpha-lipoic acid, and co-enzyme Q10), omega-3 fatty acids, curcumin, and huperzine as possible therapies for AD.

B vitamins were thought to reduce homocysteine, an amino acid suspected of playing a role in Alzheimer's. In the trial, homocysteine levels did indeed drop in the subjects who took the supplements, but it didn't change their symptoms. The study also found some evidence that the B vitamin supplements were harmful at high doses.

Researching Supplements

Scores of research studies on alternative medicine have been conducted and many more are under way. A significant number are funded, sponsored, or supported by the National Institutes of Health's National Center for Complementary and Alternative Medicine (NCCAM), an essential resource for people interested in finding reliable information about alternative medicine treatments.

NCCAM supports research on complementary and alternative medicine at universities and medical centers and spends much of its $120 million annual budget on clinical trials that put the most popular alternative treatments through the same rigorous tests the FDA requires of pharmaceuticals and medical devices.

Ⅼ Essential

Complementary care experts at the Mayo Clinic warn that herbal remedies, vitamins, and minerals, including products labeled as natural, can have druglike effects that can be dangerous. For example, the prescription coagulent Coumadin, ginkgo biloba, and vitamin E can all thin the blood. Taking these products together can increase your risk of internal bleeding or other problems.

If you are considering vitamins and other herbal remedies, be aware of the following red flags:

- If it sounds too good to be true, it probably is. You most likely cannot trust promotional materials that promise "satisfaction guaranteed," a "miracle cure," or a "startling new discovery."
- Pseudomedical and fake scientific jargon can be misleading. If a manufacturer touts a product that has been clinically tested, it may mean that one lone doctor tested a treatment. Terms such as *purify*, *detoxify*, and *energize* mean little.
- Products that claim to cure more than one complex condition, like allergies and Alzheimer's, treat a wide range of symptoms, or cure or prevent diseases are bogus.
- Absent scientific proof of health benefits, supplement manufacturers and marketers offer anecdotes and testimonials from satisfied customers: "This drug brought Mom back from the fog of Alzheimer's disease." Testimonials are not facts.
- False accusations and hints of conspiracy theories. Scam manufacturers often accuse the government or the medical

profession of suppressing important information about a product's benefits. Alzheimer's disease is a growing epidemic the government and medical profession are eager to address and treat. They have no interest in hiding information about effective treatment for AD.

Ultimately, you may choose a combination of traditional and complementary treatments to maintain health and deal with symptoms. For now, you should count on conventional medicine to diagnose your problem and treat diseases. Talk to your doctor about all treatments you pursue.

Brain Fitness

The key to building brainpower is to challenge your brain with new tasks and processes—things you've never done before, experts advise. Neurosoftware and brain games might be part of that if you like that kind of thing.

Most brain games feature memorization exercises, math problems, and pattern recognition tasks. Some test your visual attention, working memory, and reflexes. Several concentration-style memory games are based on studies of what keeps the brain active.

FIFTEEN WAYS TO PROTECT YOURSELF FROM AD

1. Dance. Ballroom dancing is best. Learning new moves stimulates motor centers in your brain and encourages new neural connections. Dancing is also a stress reducer.
2. Walk the dog—or yourself—for twenty minutes. Do it once a day, and it may lower your blood sugar.
3. Snack on almonds, not pretzels, and blueberries instead of a candy bar. The omega-3s in the almonds and the

antioxidants in the blueberries can lower your blood sugar levels and boost cognition.

4. Try walnuts instead of croutons in your salad. Walnuts, too, have omega-3s, which appear to improve mood and soothe inflammation that may lead to brain-cell death.

5. Volunteer to answer questions at the information desk at a local library, hospital, museum, or fair. Playing tour guide forces you to learn new facts and think on your feet. That helps form new neural pathways in your brain. Interacting with other people can also ease stress.

6. Try Wii or Nintendo D brain teasers

7. Move beyond your comfort zone. Good at word games? Time to move on. Brain teasers don't boost brain power once you've mastered them. Try something that doesn't come naturally: If you like numbers, learn to draw. If you love language, try logic puzzles.

8. Connect with other people to disconnect from life's many stressors: family, work, and worries.

9. Show, don't tell your brain new things. When you woke up this morning, how bright was the light in your room? What did the air smell like when you opened the window? How many colors could you discern in your garden? Pay attention to the these details to encourage prompt cell growth in the visual, verbal, and memory parts of the brain.

10. Sit quietly and choose a word that calms you. When your mind starts to wander, repeat the word to yourself. Meditation can help reduce the stress hormone cortisol, a notorious memory zapper. It also helps mitigate depression and anxiety.

11. Wear a helmet. Riding your bike is great for your health—unless you fall and get a concussion. Even one serious concussion could increase your risk of developing dementia.

12. Savor a little red wine. Drinking up to two glasses for women weekly and up to three for men delivers the anti-oxidant resveratrol, which may prevent free radicals from damaging brain cells. Sip, don't gulp. Drinking more than that could leach thiamine, a brain-boosting nutrient.

13. Check your thyroid. That tiny gland in your neck can have a effect on brain health. Thyroid hormones enhance nerve cell connections. A depleted supply of thyroid hormones may make you depressed, tired, and muddle-headed.

14. Turn up the tunes. Music soothes the savage beast, calming stress hormones that inhibit memory. Listening to music increases feelings of well-being that improve focus.

15. Plant new flowers in front of your house. Put up new pictures in the kitchen. Making such changes can alter motor pathways in the brain and encourage new cell growth.

Adapted from AARP.com, "50 Brain Boosters that Cost No Money."

Playing brain games will not restore memory loss or prevent age-related dementia, and no games marketed by reputable companies claim they will. However, experts say, the games may stimulate your brain, particularly your working memory (with which you take in and process information) and long-term memory (which stores and retrieves information).

Brain games, like most cognitive exercise, are probably more beneficial if you play them with other people. Socializing and talking uses—and may build—more brain power.

CHAPTER 7

Detecting and Diagnosing Alzheimer's

F amily members are often the first to notice the early signs of Alzheimer's: problems with memory, thinking, and language. Symptoms of early-stage AD vary from person to person, and they may seem more apparent at certain times. That is why it is important to pay attention to possible problems and keep track of how often and how regularly they occur. Any pattern should be brought to a doctor's attention. The chances of treating any disease or disorder are far better if it is detected and diagnosed in its early stages.

Signs and Symptoms: Cause for Worry?

You may notice that your gregarious dad doesn't tell his favorite stories as well as he once did—if he tells them at all. Your even-keeled mother may call you in a panic, overwhelmed because she's locked herself out of her house or lost her car in a parking garage and assumes the worst.

Write down changes you observe. This will make it much easier to see patterns, if they exist. Jot down signs of memory loss and confusion, occasions in which your loved one isn't acting like himself. Note when you first noticed the change and how long and how often it occurs.

Review the Alzheimer's Association's 10 Warning Signs from Chapter 4. If you're still not sure, ask yourself more specific questions, such as the following:

1. Is your loved one losing her spark or zest for life? Has she stopped doing things she enjoys, like going shopping with friends or taking an annual vacation?
2. Does she seem to forget things without realizing she's forgotten?
3. Is she losing judgment about money? Does she forget to pay a bill or pay it twice? Does she hand over a wallet instead of money at a checkout counter?
4. Does she start things and forget to finish them?
5. Is she talking to you less than she usually does—perhaps because she has trouble finding words?
7. Does she have difficulty organizing her thoughts and thinking clearly? Making decisions?
8. Does she get lost or disoriented in familiar places? Lose track of the time of day, days of the week, or weeks and months on the calendar?
9. Does she ask repetitive questions and seek reassurance that something will happen?
10. Does she lose things because she's misplaced them or hidden them in odd places ?
11. Is she withdrawn or apathetic? Does she seem uncharacteristically irritable or insensitive?

Source: *National Institute on Aging*

Educate yourself about Alzheimer's and other dementias. If you haven't already done so, now is the time to contact one of the reliable, go-to sources, such as the Alzheimer's Association or ADEAR, that offer information on what you need to know about Alzheimer's and other dementias.

The Value of Knowing

Incapacitating memory loss and chronic confusion are not normal indications of old age. As many as 5 to 10 percent of people who show signs of memory loss, confusion, and other symptoms of dementia may be suffering from a potentially reversible problem, such as infection, severe depression, or thyroid disease.

 Alert

The Alzheimer's Association (*www.alz.org*) operates a 24/7 hotline for questions about AD and dementia at 800-272-3900. The Alzheimer's Disease Education and Referral Center (ADEAR), part of the National Institutes of Health National Institute on Aging, offers online resources, brochures for patients and caregivers, links to clinical trials, information on studies, and more online at *www.nia.nih.gov/alzheimers* or by calling 800-438-4380.

Diagnosis can be difficult in the earliest stage of the disease, according to Eric Tangalos, MD, a primary care physician and geriatrician affiliated with the Alzheimer's Disease Research Center at Mayo Clinic. "What you're looking for is something that doesn't fit with the individual's former level of function. That's why family members often notice the symptoms first," he says. Memory loss is only one symptom of cognitive function affected by the disease. Alzheimer's can involve language, problem solving, and spatial orientation. Impaired financial skills—including problems doing simple math—are a common, under-recognized sign of early Alzheimer's disease.

Drugs approved for treatment of AD symptoms do help some people and seem to be most effective in improving quality of life in early-stage AD. Therapies to treat physical and emotional problems that can aggravate Alzheimer's may improve overall health and may even help delay some problems with cognition.

HIDING MEMORY LOSS

Portia, an independent woman in her eighties, slipped on some ice outside her apartment one January evening and was taken to a nearby hospital emergency room. Her son, John, rushed to the hospital and found his mother with a bruised wrist, impatient to go home.

The resident in charge wasn't ready to release her until he'd asked a few questions to gauge how sharp her memory was. Portia, who prided herself on her alertness, answered politely if curtly. Of course she knew her name, her address, and home phone number, she told him, and rattled off information with ease.

But when the doctor asked her who was president of the United States, she paused. Rather than risk giving the wrong answer, she changed the subject.

"I'll tell who should be president: Adlai Stevenson," she told the young physician. "Do you know who he is?" He did not.

Portia might have remembered the name of the president as soon as she left the emergency room. Or she might not have. One thing is certain: If she was experiencing progressive memory loss, she was determined not to let on.

Family Benefits

Patients and families alike are anxious about the specter of an Alzheimer's diagnosis. However, knowing that a brain disorder is the cause of your memory loss, confusion, or difficulty with speaking and writing may demystify those experiences and make them easier to manage.

Early diagnosis gives you the time to put together a medical and care team that is a good fit for you. It also gives you an opportunity to participate in studies of experimental drugs and new approaches to treatment, care, and support. Many clinical studies enroll participants in the earliest stages of the disease. Getting an early diagnosis significantly increases your chances of finding a study that might be right for you. Both drug and nondrug interventions work best in the earliest stages of Alzheimer's disease.

Question

When are most people diagnosed with Alzheimer's?
The first stage of Alzheimer's is characterized by cognitive decline, the second by functional and behavioral decline, and the third by physical decline. Most people seek diagnosis during the second stage of Alzheimer's, when they are having trouble balancing a checkbook or are getting lost.

The prospect of losing control is one of the scariest parts of an Alzheimer's diagnosis. However, being diagnosed with Alzheimer's doesn't necessarily mean you'll have to stop doing certain things, like driving a car, right away. An early diagnosis gives you more time to plan ahead and establish a routine. Early diagnosis can help you and your family understand and decide on medical, complementary, and experimental treatments. At this stage, it is important for the person who has Alzheimer's to have input. It helps if everyone who is affected by AD seeks out the best available social and emotional support.

A DIGNIFIED DIAGNOSIS

Even though he was a mental health clinician, consultant, and behavioral health care manager, Dr. Steve Hume still had to struggle to get an accurate diagnosis of early-onset Alzheimer's disease when he was sixty-one. The first neurologist Dr. Hume consulted told him he'd be fine if he just lost weight, and his frustration with the medical community has only grown since then. Far too few medical professionals know how to treat people determined to live with AD, he says.

People with Alzheimer's deserve to be treated with dignity, he says, advising patients to "tell clinicians we want a dignified diagnosis—and teach them what that means." That includes the following:

- Talk to me directly, the person with dementia.
- Tell the truth. Be honest about what you do and don't know.
- Test early. Helping me get an accurate diagnosis as soon as possible gives me more time to cope and live to my fullest potential.
- Take my concerns seriously, regardless of my age. Don't discount my concerns because I am old. At the same time, don't forget that Alzheimer's can affect people in their forties, fifties, and sixties.
- Deliver the news clearly, with consideration.
- Coordinate with my other care providers. I may have several.
- Explain the purpose of different tests and what you hope to learn from them. Testing can be very physically and emotionally challenging.
- Give me tools to live with this disease—not only medical treatment, but sources of reliable information and support.
- Work with me on a plan for healthy living.
- Recognize that I am an individual and the way I experience this disease is unique.
- Alzheimer's is a journey, not a destination. Treatment doesn't end with the writing of a prescription. Please continue to advocate—not just for my medical care but also for my quality of life.

Adapted from the Alzheimer's Association's *The Principles for a Dignified Diagnosis (co-authored by Dr. Hume)*

Making the Appointment

Schedule an appointment with a primary care doctor, internist, or family practitioner—someone who practices general medicine and knows the patient best. When you seek a diagnosis, it's very important to consult a physician who has experience with Alzheimer's and other diseases of aging. If your family doctor does not, ask her to refer you to colleagues with that expertise. Check with a local elder agency or the Alzheimer's Association for names of doctors in your area who work with these diseases.

 Fact

> Most doctors who treat people with AD are primary care physicians who are familiar with the disabilities and diseases of older people. Geriatricians and neurologists tend to be most familiar with the wide range of medical, emotional, and social needs of Alzheimer's patients and their families, but these specialists are not always available.

If your doctor suspects AD, she may refer you to a specialist for further evaluation. Alzheimer's specialists include:

- **Geriatricians:** medical doctors who specialize in the diseases, problems, and care of older age.
- **Neurologists:** physicians who specialize in diseases of the nervous system, including the brain.
- **Psychiatrists:** medical doctors who specialize in mental, emotional, and behavioral disorders.
- **Psychologists:** clinicians with advanced training in testing memory, concentration, problem solving, language, and other mental functions who sometimes evaluate people with AD and other dementias. Psychologists are not medical doctors, but they may use the title "doctor" because of their PhD degree.

Before the Doctor Visit

In this age of managed care, doctor-patient contact may be limited to less than thirty minutes per visit. For that reason, it's important to have as much information as possible with you at the appointment. That way, you don't waste half the session going over medical history and medications.

WHAT TO BRING TO A VISIT
- A list of symptoms, when they began, and when they occur
- A list of past and current medical problems and contact information for the health provider who is treating any existing condition
- A list of all current medications, including herbal and dietary supplements

Essential

Pull together a list of prescriptions and over-the-counter medications. Get doses and schedules. Update it regularly. Give copies to family members, caregivers, and health care providers. Be sure to take the list to every doctor's appointment.

Diagnosing Alzheimer's

There is no single symptom or test for Alzheimer's disease. Doctors can only confirm a diagnosis by examining brain tissue after death. But most experienced doctors can diagnose probable Alzheimer's with 90 percent accuracy based on symptoms, physical and neurological exams, and test results.

AD is diagnosed based on a process of elimination. Doctors test for other conditions that could be causing a patient's symptoms, ruling out possible diseases, disturbances, and drug interactions. They evaluate signs of other brain diseases such as vascular dementia or Lewy body dementia based on the results of tests, procedures, and exams. These include the following:

☐ **A patient health and medical history.** The doctor will want to know, what symptoms you've noticed, as well as when they began, how frequently they occur, and whether they've gotten worse. The doctor will ask about the patient's physical health, including current and past illnesses. She will ask for a family history of medical conditions, particularly if family members had Alzheimer's disease or a related disorder.

☐ **A complete physical exam.** Along with assessing overall health, most physicians will check the thyroid and look for vitamin deficiencies. They will look at symptoms of depression and other serious medical problems that can complicate diagnosis. Many older people have problems such as heart disease, diabetes, kidney disease, lung disease, or a combination of illnesses that can worsen Alzheimer's symptoms.

☐ **A neurological evaluation.** The neurological examination assesses the function of the brain and nervous system. A physician may test reflexes, coordination, and balance; muscle tone and strength; eye movement; and speech and sensation.

☐ **A mental status assessment.** A doctor will try to gauge a person's sense of time and place; the ease with which she speaks, learns, and remembers; and her ability to handle daily activities like paying bills and safely operating home appliances. Many physicians administer a brief test called the Mini Mental State Examination (MMSE) during the first office visit.

☐ **Psychiatric and neuropsychological assessments** evaluate possible symptoms of depression or other conditions that could cause cognitive problems. These tests may compare a patient's skills with those of other people of the same age, sex, and level of education. They look at different parts of the brain and brain functions to evaluate short-term and long-term memory loss, for example. Specialized evaluations look at other cognitive skills such as language, calculation, and problem solving, and can help distinguish Alzheimer's symptoms from those of other diseases such as Lewy body dementia.

❑ **Blood or urine tests** screen for certain conditions that can cause memory loss, such as anemia, thyroid problems, or vitamin deficiencies.

❑ **An electrocardiogram** checks a patient's cardiovascular health and may point to signs of vascular dementia.

❑ **Brain imaging or structural imaging tests**—magnetic resonance imaging (MRIs) or computed tomography scans (often called CAT scans or CT scans)—show the volume and shape of the brain. These tests are also used to look for signs of stroke, tumors, or head injuries, all of which can cause memory problems.

Some diagnostic workups include functional brain imaging—conducted with functional MRIs (fMRIs), positron emission tomography scans (PET scans), and single-photon emission computed tomography (SPECT scans)—that can show how well cells in various brain regions are working by showing how actively the cells use sugar or oxygen.

THE MMSE TEST

The Mini Mental State Examination (MMSE) is one of the tests most commonly used to assess mental function. A health professional asks a patient a series of questions designed to test a range of everyday mental skills, such as these:

- Remember and repeat a few minutes later the names of three common objects (for instance, horse, flower, penny)
- State the year, season, day of the week, and date
- Count backward from 100 by 7s or spell "world" backward

- Name two familiar objects present in the office as the examiner points to them
- Identify the location of the examiner's office (state, city, street address, floor)
- Repeat a common phrase or saying
- Follow a three-part instruction (for example: take a piece of paper in your right hand, fold it in half, and place it on the floor)

The maximum MMSE score is thirty points. A score of twenty to twenty-three suggests mild dementia, ten to nineteen suggests moderate dementia, and less than ten indicates severe dementia. On average, the score of an Alzheimer's patient declines by about two to four points each year.

Source: *The Alzheimer's Association*

Experts say the MMSE may not be sensitive enough to detect early memory loss in all patients, and some research indicates that highly intelligent or well-educated people score well on this test, even if they are experiencing memory loss. That is why many specialists recommend that patients undergo a neuropsychological evaluation.

Learning the Diagnosis

A diagnosis should tell you the stage of the disease and what a person is capable of doing. You should learn if there are other physical or mental ailments that could be making her memory and learning problems worse. A thorough diagnosis should help you understand basic medical, social, and psychological needs of people with AD and their loved ones, and what changes to expect in the future. Possible medical diagnoses include:

- Probable Alzheimer's disease. The doctor has ruled out other possible causes and disorders to determine that symptoms are most likely caused by Alzheimer's.
- Possible Alzheimer's disease. The doctor suspects Alzheimer's is the primary cause of signs and symptoms but may think another disease is affecting the way the disease is progressing.
- Another dementia. Physical and mental tests and symptoms suggest the patient is suffering from another degenerative disease such as vascular dementia or Lewy body dementia.
- Another disease or condition, such as a thyroid disorder, that may be reversible.

The American Psychiatric Association's *Diagnostic and Statistical Manual, Fourth Edition* (known as DSMV-IV) requires six criteria for an Alzheimer's diagnosis:

1. Evidence of memory loss and one or more of the following cognitive problems: problems with executive function (planning, organizing, sequencing); difficulty speaking or following conversations; inability to perform complex, coordinated movements such as simple physical exercises; visuospatial difficulties; staying oriented while moving through familiar surroundings.
2. Each of the problems must significantly impair work, social, or family life and indicate marked decline from her normal abilities.
3. The signs and symptoms must develop over time and gradually grow worse.
4. Medical evaluations have ruled out physical conditions such as brain tumor, stroke, and infection that can cause impairment.

5. The problems don't occur only in periods of delirium.
6. The signs and symptoms can't be explained by depression, anxiety, or other emotional disorders.

Figuring out what a person can and cannot do helps establish the right diagnosis. It also helps determine what the individual is still capable of doing either at work or at home. Physicians take into account test results and their knowledge of a patient's support system at home to gauge whether a person can still function independently or if it's time to move to a more structured, supervised environment.

Continuing Care

Following the diagnosis, you should choose a primary care physician who treats the person with AD, not the disease. You need a doctor who can monitor care, answer questions, prescribe and adjust medications, and treat other illnesses, such as diabetes and osteoporosis, that occur along with Alzheimer's.

Essential

Make sure you can count on your doctor's advice outside office hours. You will need a way to reach her or another health professional in her practice if problems arise. Make sure to find out the best way to get answers to your nonemergency questions. Can you e-mail the doctor or a nurse? Is there a help line?

Your doctor doesn't have to be a specialist; internists, family physicians, and geriatricians provide more general, comprehensive care. But your continuing care doctor should be familiar with specialists and willing to work with neurologists and psychiatrists if the need arises.

Here are some key questions about your physician to consider:

- Is the doctor able and willing to spend time with me or my loved one? (Some physicians are part of large practices that aren't set up to give doctors adequate time with patients.)
- Is she knowledgeable about patients with AD and other dementias and familiar with disease of old age?
- Is she accessible? Does the doctor or a knowledgeable associate in her practice respond to my calls and e-mails in a timely fashion?
- Can she refer me to other professionals, physical therapists, social workers, and Alzheimer's organizations?
- Does she understand and respect the role of the caregiver?

Working with Your Doctor

So what's the bottom line for successful, productive medical appointments? Ask for the information and involvement you and your family need. Plan ahead to make the best use of your time with your doctor.

Before appointments, take time to think about your loved one's symptoms and behavior; jot down precise information and observations about the person with AD so that you can answer questions during the appointment. Read up on the Alzheimer's issues that are the most important to you, such as advance directives or nursing home placement, so that you can ask questions and discuss them during the appointment. Write things down. A written list of questions can help you focus the conversation so that it covers what's important to you.

Your observations are critical to helping doctors assess your loved one's capabilities and needs. "Doctors want families to be involved," adds Dr. Tangalos of Mayo clinic. "We make better decisions when we're working closely with the people who care."

CHAPTER 8

If the Diagnosis Is Alzheimer's: First Things First

Learning that someone you love has been diagnosed with Alzheimer's disease can be upsetting and confusing, even frightening. Not only does it mean you will lose someone you care about, but it immediately thrusts you into the roles of advocate, surrogate, and caregiver. You, not your loved one, are now responsible for his medical treatment, finances, living arrangements, safety, and care. Now is a time to avoid crises: think and plan ahead.

The Big Picture

Many people are willing but few are prepared to care for a loved one with a chronic illness or degenerative brain disease. This is not a time to reinvent the wheel. Take advantage of the free, comprehensive, and accessible resources from organizations like the Alzheimer's Association (*www.alz.org*), the Family Caregiver Alliance (*www.caregiver.org*), and AARP (*www.aarp.org*). The caregiving experts at these organizations work with thousands of people and families to confront the enormous scope of the disease and the daily challenges you face. Take advantage of their advice and information, which can help guide you through unfamiliar terrain.

Gather Information

Suspecting and learning that someone you love has a degenerative brain disease can feel overwhelming. Early in the process, you may question—or deny—the diagnosis. However, your loved one is depending on you, and increasing your knowledge of Alzheimer's will help you both.

L, Essential

The Family Caregiver Alliance (FCA) offers general information, guides, and essential information on Alzheimer's disease and special needs. Much of it is published online, and some of it is available in Spanish and Chinese. It provides a wealth of resources dedicated to caregiver well-being, including training tools, communication strategies, online communities, and links to respite resources.

Write down the concerns that convinced you to seek a medical diagnosis, such as personality changes, chronic forgetfulness, or safety. This reality check can give you and the professionals you work with a big picture view of what's happening on a daily basis with the person you care for.

Educate Yourself—and Others

Talk to doctors, health and social service professionals, and people going through similar experiences. Research the disease, care, and treatment options online and in the library. Focus your research on the early and middle stages of Alzheimer's for now. The Family Caregiver Alliance provides information on:

❏ **Daily care,** including tips and advice on how to provide care and locate support services in your community.
❏ **Planning, legal, and financial advice** for Alzheimer's patients.

❏ **Living arrangements,** including information and resources on home modification and safety, housing options, and living arrangements in a care facility.

❏ **End-of-life care,** including resources on hospice and how to involve friends and family members.

Understand the Diagnosis

Alzheimer's affects each person differently, and certain symptoms and stages overlap. But common patterns occur in the progression of the illness. Knowing what those are can help you and your doctor discuss what care and treatment are best. Here are some questions you might want to ask your doctor:

❏ Can you explain why the diagnosis is Alzheimer's? What conditions of normal aging and diseases (such as severe depression) did you rule out in making the diagnosis? Why do you believe it is Alzheimer's, not another dementia or disease of old age?

❏ Are there other tests that could give us more information about the diagnosis?

❏ Should we see a medical specialist—a neurologist or psychiatrist, for example?

❏ Do you think this is early-, middle- or late-stage AD?

❏ What comes next? What symptoms should I anticipate in the next six weeks? Six months? A year from now?

❏ What is my loved one still capable of doing? Can she live on her own? Continue driving? If so, for how long? What can I do to help her maintain physical and mental health for as long as possible?

❏ Would any of the current medications for Alzheimer's symptoms be suitable now or in the future?

❏ Should we look into clinical trials?

❏ Are there nondrug therapies you know of that would help now? What about counseling, brain training, and behavior

modification programs designed to boost memory or reinforce routines?

❑ What type of routine should we follow for diet, exercise, and
staying active?

❑ What resources are available in the community for people
with AD? For families and caregivers?

Learn as much as you can about the probable progression of
your loved one's symptoms. Find out how Alzheimer's develops,
what level of care you need now, and what you are likely to need in
the months and years ahead.

Essential

Make sure you understand the specific purpose of any test the doctor mentions. Be sure you know what tests will be performed and
what they will reveal. Understand how much more you will know
once tests are completed. Ask what appointments and lab or hospital visits are involved, how long tests will take, and when you will
learn results.

Be sure to ask follow-up questions if you don't understand something. It may help to write down information so you can remember
it. That way you can discuss the diagnosis with other family members or caregivers.

Telling Others about the AD Diagnosis

A diagnosis of Alzheimer's doesn't affect just the patient.
The lives of his family members and friends may also drastically
change.

Talk with everyone involved in the patient's health and care.
Make clear that AD is a progressive brain disease, not a psychological
or emotional disorder. Like any major illness, Alzheimer's has characteristic symptoms: physical, intellectual, and behavioral changes

will occur. Encourage others to learn about those so they can better understand what lies ahead. Don't forget to discuss the diagnosis with children and teens. Encourage them to ask questions.

TALKING TO KIDS ABOUT AD

People with Alzheimer's look pretty normal, and your grandfather may not seem sick to you—at least not at first. But once you spend some time with him, you'll start to notice symptoms.

People with Alzheimer's are not crazy. They have a brain disease that damages the parts of the brain that control remembering, thinking, and feeling.

Forgetting is one of its most common symptoms. Your grandfather may forget your name—or he may call you by your sister's name, or your mother's. He might greet you with a big hug and hello in early afternoon, even though he saw you and talked to you that morning. He might ask the same questions or do something—like smoothing his hair down or tapping his fingers on a table—over and over.

At some point, he will probably have trouble finding the right words for simple things. He might point to your shoes and call them socks, for example, or forget the word *TV* and call it the "thing-a-ma-jig."

Alzheimer's disease robs people of their ability to make sense of the world. As they lose their memories, people with Alzheimer's lose the ability to do basic things, like go grocery shopping or dress for the weather. They may feel helpless. Frustrated. Angry. They may grow sad and cry. Some may act out in public in ways that embarrass the people who love them.

It's important to remember that people with Alzheimer's disease don't act like this to be mean or weird or because they don't care about you anymore. Try to understand that your grandfather's feelings for you haven't changed. He's responding to his own sadness, confusion, and frustration.

> Try to do things with your grandfather that he can still do, like setting the table or watching a ballgame. If you can, spend time with him alone, doing quiet, pleasant things. Check out the Alzheimer's Association website (*www.alz.org*) for a list of 101 activities you can do with someone with Alzheimer's disease, and a lot more information on AD.
>
> *Adapted from the Alzheimer's Association's "Living with Alzheimer's: Just for Kids."*

Assessing the Whole Patient's Needs

Discussing your loved one's diagnosis and symptoms with your doctor can help you determine what kind of assistance she will need during different phases of the illness. Every person and every situation is different. But everyone afflicted with AD eventually needs help in the following areas:

- **Health care:** medication management, physician's appointments, and physical therapy
- **Household care:** cooking, cleaning, shopping, and finances
- **Personal safety:** oversight for safety at home and to prevent wandering in early stages, round-the-clock supervision in the later stages of the disease, and assistance with transportation
- **Personal care:** bathing, eating, dressing, and grooming
- **Emotional care:** companionship, meaningful activities, and conversation

Work with a professional or use online assessment tools to put together a list of what assistance you and your loved one are likely to need. Be sure your assessment includes an evaluation of home safety and supervision. Whatever your plans for your loved one, be sure you have a reliable backup plan.

Determining Needs

Alzheimer's and geriatric specialists encourage people with AD and their families to seek a comprehensive assessment of a patient's mental, physical, environmental, and financial condition and needs. A good assessment and follow-up can help prevent accidents and illnesses, improve quality of life, and help people live in homelike environments as long as possible.

Multidisciplinary health assessments identify what a patient can and cannot do and how and what she needs to stay healthy, safe, and independent as long as possible. They provide basic but essential information—from names and doses of medications to phone numbers of family and friends—and help answer big questions about living arrangements, supervision, and assistance.

Essential

Keep a notebook and a file folder of information that you can refer back to when needed. It can include helpful articles, tip sheets, and even notes you've jotted down. Consider downloading online caregiver organizing tools from AARP, the Alzheimer's Association, or FCA.

Some hospitals and clinics offer geriatric assessments or refer patients to evaluation centers staffed by a medical team and social workers skilled in evaluating an older person's health, safety, and living situation. Independent experienced geriatric care managers can provide similar assistance, linking you and your family with services, housing, and other resources in your area. Families can complete their own assessments using standard forms from a government agency.

Coming Up with a Care Plan

Once you have an assessment, outline a comprehensive care plan that accounts for medical treatment as well as your loved one's health, safety, and comfort.

Question

What should an assessment cover?
The AARP recommends that all assessments cover physical health, mental health, medication use, the ability to live independently or with assistance, home and community safety, support system, and personal hygiene.

Line up an AD care team—partners you and your family can count on to help you provide care and comfort. It's important you have a primary care physician you trust. This person should be able to answer your questions about memory loss as well as physical and mental health. She should also be able to help you plan and arrange for health and life decisions. Your team may also include physician specialists such as geriatricians, a psychologist or clinical social worker, home health professionals, a geriatric care consultant, an elder law attorney, a counselor, and a religious or spiritual guide.

Identify Informal Help and Support

Now is the time to determine—as realistically as possible—what you are capable of, have time for, and are willing to do. Write down what you need or would like help with in the future. Include a list of informal supports—siblings, other family members, friends, and neighbors who might be able to help. You may also want to rank the advantages and disadvantages of these sources.

Fact

At this time, your loved one may be capable and independent enough to live in his own home or with a family member. He may be thriving in an assisted living or retirement community. But as his disease progresses, he will most likely need round-the-clock, skilled help with basic functions of daily living at home or in a facility. Plan and apply now.

Then, list formal services and support available in your community: community centers, adult day care, paid home health aides, and so on. Consider arranging for home-delivered meals and cleaning services and finding help with driving and other everyday activities.

Living Accommodations

Long-term care for people with dementia is expensive and in short supply in some areas of the country. Learn about the options that are available for someone with dementia. Compare them and decide which are realistic for you and your family. Find out how much care costs and what resources can help pay for it.

Assess the Current Situation

Many people are living alone or with family members when they are diagnosed with Alzheimer's, and most people prefer to remain independent. While that is understandable, it may not be safe.

To evaluate whether a home setting is the safest, most secure and comfortable place for a loved one, ask these questions:

1. Does the patient need supervision or assistance throughout the day? If so, who will provide this?
2. What activities of daily living (eating, bathing, toileting) can she perform independently? When does the doctor expect she will need more assistance?

3. Am I capable of and comfortable with providing personal care such as bathing or changing an adult diaper?
4. Can I physically, emotionally, and financially provide the care she needs?
5. Can I tap into large enough family and personal supports and professional services (such as respite care and home health services) to provide the care she needs?
6. How much outpatient medical care—doctors' appointments, physical therapy, support groups—does she need? Are those services nearby and convenient? Is transportation readily available?
7. Will she have enough pleasant, productive activity in this setting? Will she have companionship?
8. Can I make her home safe enough?

Even if you decide living at home is the best option for your loved one, look into home health care resources in your community.

What Is Home Care?

Home care is a term used to describe a range of professional, family, and community-based services that support someone recuperating from an acute injury or illness or chronic conditions, such as stroke or AD. Professionals who provide paid care in the home offer various services:

- Registered nurses (RNs) provide skilled medical care. They can give medication, monitor vital signs, dress wounds, and teach family caregivers how to use complicated equipment at home.
- Physical and occupational therapists work with patients to restore or maintain movement, speech, and cognitive skills.
- Home care aides provide personal services such as bathing, dressing, and toileting. They may also assist in making

meals, doing light housecleaning, and transporting patients to and from appointments.

- Companions/homemakers help with chores around the house and may drive and accompany a patient to activities. They do not usually provide personal care.

Line Up Essential Resources

You and your family should discuss how you will meet everyday financial responsibilities: paying bills; arranging for health, insurance, and other benefits; caring for property and investments; and preparing tax returns.

Gather information to determine your loved one's assets. Pull together bank and brokerage statements, copies of recent tax returns, social security payment information, stock and bond certificates, monthly or outstanding bills, and insurance policies. Check insurance coverage. Be aware that Medicare does not cover long-term care or custodial care.

Essential

Plan for the cost of providing long-term care for someone suffering from Alzheimer's. Calculate the cost of dementia treatment and other medical problems, such as high blood pressure, prescription drugs, and personal care items, plus the cost of adult day care, in-home care, and full-time residential care.

Line up professional advisers who can help you and your family with money matters and legal concerns. You may want to consult a geriatric care manager, who can help arrange care services, offer counseling, and see if you qualify for financial aid. Try contacting the National Association of Geriatric Care Managers (520-881-8008 or *www.caremanager.org*). Health insurance counseling is available free or at low cost to seniors. To find help in your community, call the Eldercare Locator at 800-677-1116 or visit *www.eldercare.gov*.

Getting Organized

Gather together all of your loved one's papers in one safe place. You should have certified copies of birth certificates, marriage certificates, divorce decrees, voter registration, vehicle registration and title, social security card, military identification, and discharge orders.

Alert

A person with Alzheimer's may no longer be able to drive a car, handle his own finances, or live independently in the community. But he may still have the capacity to make competent decisions about where he's going to live and what medical care and treatment he undergoes. Competent people have a moral and legal right to decide their medical treatment.

Put together a list of your loved one's financial assets and liabilities: checking and savings accounts, social security income, certificates of deposit, stocks and bonds, real estate deeds, insurance policies and annuities, retirement or pension benefits, credit card debts, home mortgages and loans, and so forth. Try to keep copies of records in one or two places, such as a bank safety deposit box and a home file cabinet. Start a ledger of income and expenses; keep records of when money comes in and bills are due. Think about opening an online bank account to pay bills.

Prepare for Change

Many families reject the idea of moving a loved one to a nursing home at any point. They believe a family setting is the best place to assure a loved one's health, safety, and happiness. But experts say that isn't always the case.

"I promised my parents I'd never put them in a nursing home." It's something Joanne Koenig Coste, author of *Learning to Speak Alzheimer's*, hears all the time. "Yes, you promised," she answers. "But they didn't promise they'd never have Alzheimer's. There are good places out there. Nursing homes aren't at all what they used to be. Some have great programs. Many Alzheimer's people actually seem to do better when they're placed."

Essential

Take advantage of free online tools such as the AARP's caregiving checklists for evaluating assisted living and nursing home facilities. You can find and download them at *http://assets.aarp.org/external_sites/ caregiving/options/nursing_homes.html*. AARP also provides helpful information on calculating the differences in costs of independent living, assisted living, and long-term care.

The national Alzheimer's Disease Education and Referral Center (ADEAR) recommends asking these questions and discussing them with a doctor or another knowledgeable professional who can help you determine if your loved one can continue living on her own or in a relatively unsupervised setting.

DOES THE PERSON WITH AD:
❑ Become confused or unpredictable under stress?
❑ Recognize a dangerous situation, such as a fire?
❑ Use the telephone in an emergency?
❑ Know the fastest, most efficient ways to get help?
❑ Generally stay content within the home?
❑ Wander and become disoriented?
❑ Show signs of agitation, depression, or withdrawal when left alone for any period of time?
❑ Try to pursue interests or hobbies like cooking or woodworking that might now need supervision?

If you answered yes to any of those questions, it may be time for a change, according to health and safety experts at ADEAR.

Alzheimer's experts say a change in your loved one's living situation is mandatory if she has experienced severe weight loss in the past six months, can't take medications on schedule, visited the emergency room or doctor frequently, cannot remember to buy new food, or wanders outside the home.

Fact

Senior Housing Finder, powered by SNAPforSeniors, provides detailed listings of licensed residences throughout the United States that offer services especially for residents with dementia. Its information is objective and easy to search. It currently lists more than 65,000 licensed facilities. Visit *www.snapforseniors.com* to find one near you.

Long-Distance Caregiving

Even if you live far away, there's a lot you can do to help your loved one in our wireless, digital age. More than 7 million American adults provide long-distance care to aging relatives who live more than an hour away, according to the National Institute on Aging (*www.nia.nih.gov*). The federal agency's excellent guide, *So Far Away: Twenty Questions for Long-Distance Caregivers*, suggests skills and strategies to help. Some are adapted here:

1. **When you can't lend a hand, lend an ear.** Check in regularly with your loved one and his caregiver. Hearing a familiar, friendly voice can mean a lot to both of them on tough days. Help your loved one stay in touch. Program his phone with important phone numbers—yours, other family members', the doctor's. Be prepared for the fact that a loved one with dementia may call you repeatedly, several times a day. Decide how you will handle this if it happens to you.

2. **Always connect.** Get in touch with neighbors, family, friends, and others who live close by. Tell them what's going on and make sure they know how to reach you if necessary. Put together a phone book that includes contact information for family, close friends, doctors, caregivers, and all resources for elders and people with dementia in your loved one's community.

3. **Learn what you need to know about the disease, condition, and treatment plan.** Understand the progression of dementia and find out as much as you can about your loved one's current symptoms and condition. Learn how he, his doctor, and his caregiver are managing the illness. Nothing frustrates caregivers so much as family members who live far away and don't make an effort to understand the difficulties of dealing with AD from day to day.

4. **Offer help, not advice.** Listen to what the caregiver says and doesn't say. If she's overwhelmed or having difficulty, don't offer your opinion or suggestions about solving the problem. Find help! Get online, research support services, and find some solutions.

5. **Deal with details.** Gather information, set up systems, and take care of tasks. You can pay your loved one's bills, do his taxes, research long-term care facilities, and track clinical trials online. Virtual help can be extremely valuable to families living with AD.

6. **When you can't spend time, send money to help with the expense of day-to-day care.** Consider hiring someone who can take over for the caregiver a few hours each week.

7. **Plan family visits.** Plan your visits to help make your loved one's life a little brighter and the caregiver's burden lighter. Talk to your family members ahead of time to see what help they need. Then make clear, realistic plans to get some of that done. Try to give family members who live close by a break from care and a chance to do the things

they don't have time for—talking to a social worker or taking Mom shopping, for example. Be sure to spend time visiting with your loved one and enjoying one another's company while you're there.

⌷ Essential

Make sure at least one family member has written permission to receive medical and financial information. Try putting together a notebook that includes all the vital information about health care, social services, and contact numbers.

Long-distance caregivers may find the following titles from the National Institute on Aging of particular interest:

- **Home Safety for People with Alzheimer's Disease**
  (*www.nia.nih.gov/alzheimers/publications/homesafety.htm*)
- **Good Nutrition: It's a Way of Life**
  (*www.niapublications.org/agepages/nutrition.asp*)
- **Older Drivers**
  (*www.nia nih.gov/healthinformation/publications/drivers*)
- **Caregiver Guide: Tips for Caregivers of People with Alzheimer's Disease**
  (*www.nia.nih.gov/alzheimers/publications/caregiver guide.htm*)
- **Nursing Homes: Making the Right Choice**
  (*www.niapublications.org/agepages/longterm.asp*)

The NIA provides many helpful resources for patients with Alzheimer's disease families, and caregivers.

CHAPTER 9

If You Have Alzheimer's Disease

If you've been diagnosed with Alzheimer's disease, you may be shocked, angry, anxious, or depressed. You may think this can't be true for you. These reactions are normal. Remember, though, that you are neither your diagnosis nor your disease. Many people with AD continue to live full lives. Doing that involves some learning, thinking, and planning. Understanding your illness—and how others with AD cope with theirs—can help you stay healthy, safe, independent, and happy as long as possible.

Talking with Your Doctor

A good doctor cares not only about your medical condition, but your general health and well-being as well. Here are some questions you may want to ask about your diagnosis:

- What kind of changes should I expect over the next six to twelve months?
- Would any of the current medications for Alzheimer's symptoms be suitable for me now or in the future?
- If I start taking medication, what kind of improvements and side effects can I expect?
- Should I consider participating in a clinical trial for Alzheimer's treatments?

- What nondrug therapies and support do you recommend?
- What advice do you have regarding diet, exercise, and staying active?
- What resources are available in the community for people with AD?
- Is there educational information you can give me? What online education and support resources do you recommend?
- Can I call you—or someone in your practice—with questions between appointments?

Never hesitate to ask your doctor, nurse, or other health care provider to repeat any instructions or medical terms you don't understand or remember. They should always be available to answer your questions and address your concerns.

Alert

People in early-stage Alzheimer's often feel misunderstood because myths and misconceptions about the disease have created a stigma about it. Remember: people with early-stage AD are living with Alzheimer's, not dying from it.

Before each appointment, try to make a list of questions for your doctor or someone in his practice. Always take someone you trust with you to your appointments. Ask your companion to take notes and help explain anything you don't understand.

First Responses

After receiving a diagnosis, you might want to deny you have dementia. You may fear losing people who are important to you and feel lonely, because no one seems to understand what you're going through. It's frustrating when you can't do things as easily as you have before, or if you have difficulty making yourself understood.

Find out as much as you can about AD. Talk to loved ones and other people you trust. No one understands this as much as other people living with AD. No one understands what you're going through as well as other people with AD and the people who support them. Learn about services and support resources for people with AD, and consider joining a support group—online, in your community, or both.

SUPPORT GROUPS

"That touchy-feely stuff is not for me!" Ken told his doctor when he suggested Ken consider joining an early-stage Alzheimer's support group. Now, Ken says, "I don't know what I'd do without my group!"

Ken meets once a week with eight to ten other people living with early-stage Alzheimer's, who offer one another emotional support, practical information, and tips on how to cope with their disease. They meet on Friday mornings at a local community health center, where a social worker leads discussions and helps individual members connect with services (like transportation) they might need.

Some support groups are more formal and structured than Ken's, led by an expert whose role is to educate the group. Others are less formal get-togethers of people who share a common concern—often an illness, like AD or cancer—and who take turns leading discussions.

Not everyone wants or needs support from people other than family and friends. But many, like Ken, feel that other people in his situation offer special help in dealing with the disease.

"A lot of us want to live as normally [as we can] as long as we can. But my life is different from my friends—most of them are still working—and from other people's. People treat you differently when they know you have Alzheimer's. They think you're stupid, not just slow at certain things. The only people who really understand that are other people with the disease."

People who don't have easy access to group meetings—or don't care for them—sometimes join online support groups. There are an increasing number of message boards, chat rooms, and blogs for people with Alzheimer's. Check the Alzheimer's Association website (*www.alz.org*) to find virtual support from people like you.

Essentials

Alzheimer's is demanding and tiring. The simple tasks of daily living take longer. You find you can't do certain things you like to do, or are used to doing yourself. You can't count on your memory, and you may feel confused, disoriented, and incapable of making sound decisions. These physical and emotional changes are frustrating and can be disheartening. They can damage your self and self-esteem, which is why it is essential that you maintain your physical and emotional health. Follow these tips to bolster positive feelings:

- Treat yourself with care and respect.
- Eat regularly and well.
- Exercise (with your doctor's approval) every day. You don't have to go to the gym. Go for a walk. Garden. Get outdoors.
- Take your medications on schedule. Get help organizing pills and setting up reminder systems if you need to.
- Continue doing things you like to do, such as swimming or gardening.
- Spend time with people you care about, do things you enjoy.
- If you drink alcohol, cut back. Drinking can diminish your memory and thinking abilities.
- Avoid situations, tasks, or activities that cause you anxiety.
- Watch out for depression and stress.
- Rest when you're tired.
- When you feel anxious or overwhelmed, take a break.

Coping with Your Symptoms

Knowledge is power. If you know what to expect as you live with AD, you can cope better with symptoms as they develop.

Essential

Because you are dealing with a brain disease, it's essential that you limit your risk for falls and accidents. Ask your doctor to review your medications to see if any might affect your balance. Always use a seat belt in a vehicle, and be a careful pedestrian. Put on protective head gear if you bicycle or engage in sports.

Memory Loss

You may forget people's names or what something is called. Your memory of the past may be just fine, but you have trouble recalling things that happened recently—even earlier today. Memory problems are a common symptom of AD. Consider these tried and tested recommendations from others who've learned to cope with these common problems:

❏ Make a book of important information, such as your name, address, and emergency contact information. Use it to keep track of people's names and contact information. Keep a list of your appointments. Use the book to write down thoughts, ideas, and memories you want to hold on to.

❏ Put sticky notes around the house when you need to remember things.

❏ Leave written reminders to yourself like, "Turn off the stove" or "Unplug the iron." Be sure you have an automatic shut-off feature on the appliances you use most often, especially the ones that can cause harm if left unattended.

❑ Label cupboards and drawers with words or pictures of their contents.

❑ Place important phone numbers in large print next to the phone.

❑ Tack up a schedule of things you do daily. Include meal times, exercise, and medication times.

❑ If it helps, have someone call to remind you of important things that you need to do at certain times during the day, like meal times, medication times, and appointments.

❑ Label photos of people you see often.

❑ Keep track of phone messages with voice mail or an answering machine.

❑ Use whatever memory aids work: a pocket notepad, personal digital assistant, wristwatch alarm, or voice recorder can help you remember what you have to do or keep track of information.

Communication Problems

AD affects language as well as memory. You may start talking to someone and forget what you're talking about when you're halfway through a sentence. You might forget words and names.

Question

What can I do if I keep losing things?
Put things you tend to lose a lot in the same spot. Choose a place for glasses, keys, your hearing aids, and anything you're prone to misplacing. Always put them in that spot when you're not using them.

Remember to take your time. Take a break if something is too difficult. And keep on talking! People who socialize even once a day preserve their memories longer than those who don't, studies say.

Disorientation

You may have trouble keeping track of days of the week and time. You may find yourself going to a lunch date a day early or late, or forget where you said you would meet someone. You might go for a walk on a glorious day and find you're lost. The following suggestions will help you deal with these issues:

- Cross off days on the calendar to keep track of time.
- Take someone with you when you go out.
- Keep a map with you or use a GPS device.
- Don't be afraid to ask for help. If you explain to others that you have a memory problem and need assistance, they are almost certain to give you a hand.

Spatial Perception Problems

AD affects physical coordination and your sense of distance between things. You might have trouble climbing stairs because you misjudge their height. You may also find yourself bumping into familiar objects in your home. Some people have trouble getting out of cars or putting on a coat. Allow yourself the time to do the things you need to do, and don't feel rushed or let other people rush you.

Essential

Talk to yourself. Say words out loud. Saying "I've turned off the oven" as you shut it off will give you an extra verbal reminder when you later try to recall whether you left it on. Repeating names when you're introduced to someone has the same effect.

Visual Perception

You might look straight at a cell phone and forget what it's used for, or hand a cashier your wallet when you meant to give him dollar bills. You may "lose" things in the drawers and cupboards of your home. Take your time. Take breaks. Try not to get upset.

Problems with Reasoning and Judgment

AD sometimes affects common sense about things like what clothing is appropriate for the day and season. It can cause absent-mindedness and mishaps; some people find they regularly do things like lock themselves out of the house. Others find they are bothered all day by a problem they forget to discuss, then later that problem turns into an obsession.

Most problems have solutions. Have someone help you sort through your closets and drawers, or ask a family member to do it. Leave a set of house keys with a neighbor you trust. Schedule chats with family, friends, or someone in your community each day. Keep a list of things you want to discuss.

KEEPING TRACK

Why ask someone with memory loss to use a calendar? Because it helps proactive patients function and feel better.

"Training yourself to use a calendar is kind of like driving a stick shift or typing on a computer keyboard," says Sherrie Hanna, a program coordinator at Mayo Clinic in Rochester, Minnesota, where researchers are studying the effectiveness of memory training workshops and tools. "You don't think about all the motions involved in the process. You don't say to yourself, 'Okay, now I'm going to depress the clutch with my left foot and move the shifter with my right hand.' You just do it."

"Just doing it" helps proactive patients with early-stage memory loss hang on to a sense of independence and accomplishment. Patients in Hanna's six-week workshops learn to use monthly pocket calendars to write down scheduled events, daily "to-do-today" lists, and anything else that strikes them as important, from the weather to a phone number to the fact that grapes are on sale this week.

"Writing something down in a calendar helps it stick in your memory," Hanna says. "Saying it out loud as you're writing it down also can help cement it in your memory." Using colors, pictures, and other sensory aids can help even more.

Hanna encourages people to check their calendars twice a day. "Three times is even better. We also tell them to check things off right when they do it. So even if they don't remember doing something—if it's checked off, they must have done it."

In the early stages of memory loss, "many people feel the control slipping out of their fingers," she says. Having information on hand gives people a sense of responsibility and control over day-to-day life.

Coping with Your Feelings

When you are diagnosed, you may be shocked or go into denial. That's normal. You'll probably feel angry. Sadness and frustration are part and parcel of the disease. If you're like most people, you will sometimes feel depressed or angry that your life is changing. You'll worry, and you'll wonder if you're losing your sense of self.

Fact

People living with AD recommend finding out as much as you can about the illness and talking to your friends and family about it. Don't isolate people. You will need them, and they will want to be involved in helping to take care of you.

The feelings you may be experiencing are normal. But it is important to find ways to deal with depression, anxiety, and stress. Depression makes AD symptoms worse. Prolonged stress can lead to frustration, anger, hopelessness, and depression. Stress affects you, your family, and anyone who cares about you or for you.

Talk to your physician, who can determine if there is an appropriate treatment for feelings you find overwhelming. Talk to a counselor, a clergy member, or someone with whom you can share your spiritual needs. Share your feelings with your friends and family or a support group.

Sharing Your Diagnosis

As you come to recognize that your diagnosis is real—that you will live with AD for the rest of your life—you will probably want people you love and care for to know about your disease. Telling people you have AD is not easy. Even if you've begun to come to grips with your diagnosis, sharing it with someone you love may make it seem more "real," even threatening—particularly if the other person is surprised or very upset by your news.

Essential

Once you retire, be sure to find a volunteer activity or hobby that will take the place of your job. Retirement is a major change and challenge for most people. It's particularly important that you have retirement plans in place when you're dealing with AD.

Consider who you want to tell and how and when to tell them. You may want to discuss this with your doctor, caregiver, or with other people who have AD. Start with the people closest to you—people you'd tell about any illness or major change in your life. These are people with whom you're comfortable, people you trust.

You don't have to tell people everything about your illness, though it may help you to have some information about Alzheimer's to help explain the disease and what to expect as it progresses.

You can ask someone you trust to help you talk to others about your AD diagnosis.

Your friends and neighbors want to know how you are doing. Talk to them. Stay in touch. If you're like most people, you probably don't like asking others for help. Remember: Most people who care about other people want to help in any way they can.

Keeping Track of Money and Vital Records

Many people with AD have trouble keeping track of basic money matters—what checks they've written and bills they've paid. You might do this. And you may wake up at night, worrying about whether you have enough money, whether your will is up to date, or what will happen if you are too ill to communicate.

As soon as possible after your diagnosis, talk with your family. Make plans—and make your wishes known now, so your family can honor them in the future.

Arrange for direct deposits of checks, such as your retirement pension or social security benefits. Make sure your money matters will be in the hands of someone you trust. Talk to a lawyer about naming someone to look after your financial interests.

Fact

Joining an early-stage support group can help you and your family learn about Alzheimer's and get useful advice about living with dementia. A support group can also help you connect with people who know and understand your situation best, because they've confronted the symptoms you face and the anxiety, sadness, anger, or fear that you might be experiencing.

You may want to appoint a substitute decision maker who can act on your behalf when you are very ill. Even if you choose not to write things down or draw up a legal document, it's important to talk about these matters. Let those closest to you know what you want and what you do not want for your future health and personal care.

Steps for Getting Your Affairs in Order

❑ Gather everything you can about your income, property, investments, insurance, and savings.

❑ Put copies of legal documents and other important papers in one place. You could set up a file, put everything in a desk or dresser drawer, or just list the information and location of papers in a notebook.

❑ If your papers are in a bank safe deposit box, keep copies in a file at home. Check regularly to see if there's anything new to add.

❑ Tell a trusted family member or friend where you put your important papers. You don't need to tell this person your personal business, but someone should know where you keep your papers in case of an emergency.

❑ If you don't have a relative or friend you trust, ask a lawyer to help.

Source: *ADEAR*

Live the Life You Lead Well

If you've been diagnosed with AD and you are reading this, you are probably a resourceful, proactive, intelligent person concerned about health, safety, and quality of life. Illness is stressful, anxiety-producing, and sometimes depressing. Enlist the help of loved ones and caregivers to cut down on the anxieties of day-to-day living. Get help organizing your life so you can save energy and reduce stress.

Get help with grocery shopping and planning meals. Consider having groceries and prepared foods delivered, or buy frozen prepared meals. Hire someone to clean your house and take care of your yard.

More and more resources are available to help people with early-stage dementia cope with their feelings and the practical aspects of everyday living. And more and more people with Alzheimer's are sharing advice on how to improve your quality of life.

This is what many of them advise: Don't forget to relax and enjoy life. Watch funny movies. Listen to music. Try something new. Spend time with pets. Make plans and go out with friends and family. Keep busy and active. Try helping others. Dance. Sing. And don't forget to laugh.

CHAPTER 10

Staying Safe and Secure with AD

People living with AD gradually lose the ability to think and reason, to judge what is or isn't practical and safe. Even if your loved one is alert and relatively independent, you should take precautions now to help keep her safe and secure for as long as possible. It is essential that you anticipate the time when it is no longer safe for her to live alone. Experts advise that long before the need arises, you should plan for full-time professional help or for moving her to an eldercare facility.

The Car Key Conundrum

Adult children would rather talk to their parents about funeral plans than about giving up their car keys, according to a survey conducted by the National Safety Council and Caring.com, an online site for baby boomers caring for their parents. One-fourth of the adult children surveyed said they would like to see their elderly parents limit their driving. Some 33 percent favored some type of mandatory testing or restrictions on elderly drivers.

When your mom scoffs at your suggestion that she give up her car—she insists she's safe, because she drives slowly and not very far or very often—she may have a point. If she's physically healthy and in early-stage dementia, she may not pose a danger to herself or others right now.

Driving a car is a complex activity that demands quick reactions, alert senses, and split-second decision-making. Most people are aware that normal aging impairs vision, limits physical mobility, and slows reaction time. Many older people drive less than they once did, of their own volition. They may also drive more slowly and avoid driving at night. Evidence suggests that many older drivers are wiser drivers.

🗒 Fact

Baby boomers point out frequently that elderly drivers have more accidents than any other group of drivers except teenagers. Statistics on current road deaths show that people over the age of sixty-five are 16 percent more likely to cause accidents than those age twenty-five to sixty-four. Drivers under twenty-five are 188 percent more likely to cause crashes than are middle-aged adults.

However, because AD and other dementias diminish judgment, many people with the conditions continue to drive as their symptoms grow worse, posing a danger to themselves, their passengers, and the community at large. Others simply fail to recognize declining abilities or dread the prospect of giving up driving, fearing it will isolate them or make them utterly dependent on others for the necessities of life.

Be proactive and discuss the possibility of giving up driving with your loved one before it becomes an emergency. Come up with a plan for allowing her to get around and get groceries and other necessities when she is no longer able to drive. Friends and family may be able to help out, and there may be public transportation or shuttle services you can look into.

Addressing Driving Dilemmas

The AARP has compiled a list of warning signs that can help you assess whether it's time to limit or give up driving. They include:

1. Feeling uncomfortable and nervous or fearful while driving.
2. Dents and scrapes on the car or on fences, mailboxes, garage doors, curbs, or other objects. Recent tickets for traffic or parking violations.
3. Difficulty staying in the lane of travel.
4. Getting lost.
5. Trouble paying attention to signals, road signs, and pavement markings.
6. Slower response to unexpected situations. Frequent close calls.
7. Medical conditions or medications that may be affecting the ability to handle the car safely.
8. Other drivers honking at you and instances when you are angry at other drivers.
9. Friends or relatives not wanting to drive with you.
10. Being easily distracted or having a hard time concentrating while driving.

If you notice one or more of these warning signs, visit the AARP website (*www.aarp.org/families/driver_safety*) for comprehensive information and advice on senior driving. Consider having a professional assess driving skills. Consult a doctor.

Meanwhile, try to be as understanding and objective as possible about what giving up driving really means to a driver. Ride with her to observe her driving habits firsthand.

When you talk about driving, make clear you're concerned about her health and well-being, and base what you say on things you know (her grandchildren don't want to ride with her) or have observed (two traffic violations in the past year).

Suggest various options, depending on the degree of her impairment. One size does not fit all; while stopping driving may be the only answer in some cases, stopping driving too early can cause a person's overall health to decline prematurely, warns the AARP.

Some people are so threatened or upset by the prospect of giving up their freedom to drive that they continue to ignore the advice and admonitions of their families, physicians, and friends. Check out *www.seniordrivers.org*, sponsored by the American Automobile Association Foundation for Traffic Safety. The site features online tips and guides to seniors on driving safely and information and advice for families that can help everyone plan ahead for a time when driving is no longer safe. Just as important, it offers information on alternative transportation for seniors in their communities.

Question

But what if no one close by can drive my mother?
Look into the cost of hiring taxicabs, shuttle services, and independent drivers. Before you dismiss the idea of spending money on transportation needs, tally up the cost of buying gas, car insurance, and maintaining a car each year. Compare that to the price of hiring a driver to take your mother to and from her home. You may actually save money.

If you've tried all sensible solutions to deal with the issue and none have worked, consider these suggestions from the National Institute on Aging.

- If your loved one drives against her doctor's advice, ask the doctor to write to the Department of Motor Vehicles or Department of Public Safety saying she should no longer drive.
- Ask the doctor for a prescription that says your loved one cannot drive.

Staying Safe at Home

As AD progresses, some people experience personality and behavior changes and do things that may endanger themselves. Many people with dementia, for example, wander from home and become lost at some point. Some, confused about the difference between day and night, wake up, get dressed, and start to leave the house in the middle of the night, thinking the day has just started. Many suffer losses of hearing, vision, taste, or smell. They don't hear phones or smell what's burning in the oven.

Question

How can I encourage my loved one to give up driving gradually?
Ask him to look into other means of transportation: getting rides, using public transit, calling cabs, or hiring a driver. Urge him to try out a few. Be sure you or someone responsible goes with him when he tries out local buses or car services.

The Alzheimer's Disease Education and Referral Center advises that you modify the home environment:

- Display emergency numbers and your home address near all telephones. Use an answering machine or voice mail to answer phone calls and set it to turn on after the fewest number of rings possible. A person with AD may become unable to take messages. Be wary of telephone exploitation and fraud. Turn ringers on low to avoid distraction and confusion.
- Install smoke alarms near all bedrooms and carbon monoxide detectors in appropriate places; check their functioning and batteries frequently.
- Install secure locks on all outside doors and windows.
- Hide a spare house key outside in case the person with AD locks you out of the house.
- Avoid clutter, which can create confusion and danger. Limit use of extension cords, placing lamps and appliances close to electrical outlets. Tack extension cords to the baseboards to avoid tripping.

- Cover unused outlets with childproof plugs.
- Place red tape around floor vents and radiators.
- Put away heating pads and electric blankets.
- Throw out or recycle newspapers and magazines regularly. Keep all walk areas free of furniture, scatter rugs, and space heaters.
- Keep plastic bags out of reach.
- Lock up all power tools and machinery.

Safety Outside

Be sure to safety-proof outdoors as well. Keep steps sturdy and textured to prevent falls in wet or icy weather. Mark the edges of steps with bright or reflective tape. Think about installing a ramp with handrails at an entrance to the home rather than using steps. Eliminate uneven surfaces, walkways, hoses, planters, or other objects that may cause someone to trip.

In addition, you should restrict access to a swimming pool by fencing it in. Put away your gas grill and any fuel sources or fire starters when they're not in use. Be sure to supervise any time anyone in the household uses the grill.

Medications

Be sure to keep all prescription and over-the-counter medicine in one place. Label each prescription medicine with the patient's name, name of the drug, drug strength, dosage frequency, and expiration date. Use sorters and pill reminders to keep track of daily doses.

Alcohol and Cigarettes

You should keep all alcohol in a locked cabinet or out of reach of the person with AD. Drinking alcohol can increase confusion. If someone in the household smokes, remove matches, lighters, ashtrays, and cigarettes from view. This will reduce fire hazards. It may also encourage someone with Alzheimer's who smokes to quit or cut down, smoking only when someone else is present.

Money and Fraud Protection

People who are in the early stages of Alzheimer's disease frequently have difficulty writing out a check or reading a bank statement. Even patients with few noticeable AD symptoms may have trouble paying bills or counting change, according to Daniel Marson, director of the Alzheimer's Disease Center at the University of Alabama–Birmingham.

Because AD affects judgment, people with the illness are more likely to be taken in by fraud schemes, says Marson. While most healthy seniors he has studied had no trouble recognizing suspicious signs in a letter outlining a financial scam, many Alzheimer's patients were duped or swayed by the letter.

Essential

According to Marson, warning signs of increased confusion about money matters include forgetting to pay bills or paying more than once, problems keeping track of finances or bills, making mistakes in math and counting in everyday life, difficulty understanding basic financial terms, and a new interest in get-rich-quick schemes.

That's why phone and mail fraud schemes often target the elderly. "Patients lose the ability to size up the situation," Marson told *USA Today*. "And before you know it, they've made a sizable donation."

Pay attention to basic consumer protection for people with AD. Seniors spent some $4.5 billion on bank overdraft fees in 2007, according to the Center for Responsible Lending, a nonprofit, nonpartisan research and policy organization. More and more elderly people are switching over to debit cards after years of relying on checkbooks and cash, and many are unfamiliar with how debit card deposits, purchases, and cash advances work. They don't know when electronic deposits or withdrawals will hit their accounts. Consider setting up online access to the account so that caregivers and people with AD can easily monitor account balances and see which checks, debits, and deposits have cleared.

Besides raising routine fees, banks now engage in practices that make it easier to overdraw accounts, such as holding deposits longer than necessary, according to the research group. Bank fees add up quickly, particularly for seniors on fixed incomes, and they can decimate monthly budgets.

Continuing Care Communities

There will likely come a time when someone with AD needs more care and supervision than you can provide outside a specialized eldercare setting. As you begin to look into long-term care for your loved one, familiarize yourself with some of the key terms used in the world of eldercare.

Knowing the differences between independent living, assisted living, and long-term care is critical to finding and evaluating what's best for anyone with AD. Be aware that the terms for housing options for older adults vary from state to state. There is no standard national definition for "assisted living," for example. In many areas, it refers to semi-independent living, often in an eldercare complex, and usually with on-site assistance. But in some states, where assisted living is not licensed or regulated, the term may be used very loosely, describing facilities that offer few of the services many people expect with assisted living.

Older people's needs often change over time, and many eldercare facilities called they are set up to address those changing needs. These facilities, sometimes called eldercare communities, tend to be well-designed, safe, and secure. There's a wide variation in what continuing care communities provide, but most offer a range of options, from independent living units to assisted living to skilled nursing facilities, all in one place. Be aware, though, that these facilities can be extremely expensive. Many will care for residents as their needs change.

Fact

Most continuing care communities offer different levels of on-site care at different costs. If a resident suddenly needs more assistance or intensive nursing care, it's available on site. But it may not be as readily or easily available as families assume. Many independent living facilities are not licensed to provide ongoing medical care, and their contracts seldom cover special services. If your loved one needs more care or help, you may have to arrange and pay for the services, which are available elsewhere on site.

These tend to be well designed, safe, and secure. They offer different levels of on-site care at different costs. If a resident suddenly needs more assistance or intensive nursing care, it's available on site. However, most continuing care facilities are extremely expensive. Most charge an entrance fee and some require that you purchase an apartment or condominium before moving in.

Independent Living Facilities

In most cases, these are apartments within a continuing care complex, designed for people who are essentially healthy but may need some assistance for themselves or a spouse. They tend to offer on-site amenities such as banks, fitness programs, communal meals, and beauty salons. Some offer on- and off-site adult education classes and cultural activities.

Assisted Living Facilities

Assisted living is a broad term for housing for people who can no longer live independently but don't need assistance or complex medical care on a daily basis. Typically, the facilities offer a room or small apartment and meals, along with personal care and support services, social activities, and twenty-four-hour supervision.

Families often believe that assisted living facilities can meet all of their loved ones' needs: meals, household help, transportation, and assistance with daily living and medical care when necessary. Many assisted living facilities, however, are not legally allowed to provide medical care.

Alert

The federal government doesn't regulate assisted-living facilities, and state regulations vary—as does the level and quality of service at each facility. In some places, unlicensed staff provide most resident care, including administration of medication. Adequate nursing care and supervision is essential to the health and safety of anyone with dementia and other chronic diseases.

While assisted living may seem like an excellent solution for an elder who needs a little help, most people with AD need much more. Assisted living "is not an option for people whose illnesses are so debilitating that they're unable to leave their beds, or for people suffering from severe cases of dementia," say eldercare experts at AARP. Some assisted living facilities now offer special units for patients with Alzheimer's disease.

Skilled Nursing or Long-Term Care Facilities

These specialized facilities provide round-the-clock medical care, usually administered by registered nurses and aides under the supervision of doctors. Many offer physical, speech, and occupational therapy, as well as assistance with activities of daily living. Some specialize in dementia and Alzheimer's care.

Starting Your Search

If you're considering a group setting for someone with AD and you know your preferred location, consider contacting the federal government's eldercare locator at 800-677-1116 or visiting *www. eldercare.gov*. The eldercare locator will put you in touch with the appropriate Area Agency on Aging (AAA), whose staff keeps vital information about the availability and basic quality of group housing facilities in your area. AAA staff members know all about state licensing and regulatory requirements, ways to obtain information about specific facilities, and which facilities accept people whose costs are paid by Medicaid.

Once you've got a list of facilities recommended by an AAA (or from the Alzheimer's Association), call each one. AARP warns that you should remember that the person you speak with will most likely be a marketing or salesperson whose job it is to sell you a contract.

Make sure you ask and get answers to the questions that are most important to you and, if you're interested, that you ask the representative to send brochures and details including a price list, a map or floor plan, a list of the residents' rights and rules, and copies of all the documents you will be required to sign before your loved one moves in, including the contract.

NURSING HOME RATINGS

You can check out Medicare's ratings of 16,000 nursing homes at Nursing Home Compare, an interactive online tool at *www .medicare.gov/nhcompare*. Using its own agency data and a five-star rating system, Medicare assigns rankings to facilities in three categories—health inspections, staffing levels, and quality measures—to calculate overall ratings.

In 2008, 12 percent of nursing homes earned five-star ratings, and 22 percent earned only one star. Approximately 35 percent of the facilities received three-star ranks or higher, according to AARP.com.

Health care advocates applaud the rating system as a useful tool that can help consumers quickly find out which homes to avoid. But they caution that the ratings should be viewed and used selectively.

Unlike a five-star restaurant or hotel, a five-star rating is not a guarantee of overall high quality, eldercare advocates told AARP.com. Medicare's ratings are based on staff and quality measurement data that the nursing homes report themselves and are not independently confirmed. Nor do the ratings indicate how many staff are skilled professionals and how many are temporary workers who may not deliver the same quality of care. AARP recommends that you visit nursing homes, talk to doctors and people you trust, and check state assessments of nursing home inspections before you choose a long-term care facility.

Visiting and Evaluating Facilities

Take your questions and a checklist with you when you visit the facility. Pay attention to your gut feeling and notice what is going on around you as staff guide you on a tour, which is sure to highlight the most appealing aspects of the facility. Chat with staff. Talk to residents. Try to visit more than once. "An unscheduled visit on a weekend or in the evening might be very helpful in making your decision," say AARP experts.

L. Essential

Ask your local AAA which facilities are licensed and under what rules. Don't even think about a place that isn't licensed. If you want more information, a state licensing agency office can tell you if there have been any complaints filed against any of the facilities on your list. After all, having a state license doesn't assure quality care.

AARP advises that you wait before signing a contract. Take it home, read it again, and go over it with the rest of the family. Seek professional legal or financial advice if you are concerned about any part of the contract. The contract outlines the specific responsibilities the facility will provide to your loved one. If it isn't in the contract, it isn't part of the services your loved one will receive.

Be sure to compare details in your contract with what's touted in the sales brochure. Scrutinize fees, the overall level of care, and the health care services in particular. Make sure the amenities touted in the brochure are included and described in detail in the contract.

Remember, you are almost sure to feel uneasy, frustrated, and overwhelmed as you search for the best living situation for a loved one. Keep in mind that the best choice is the one that best suits your loved one's health, social, and financial needs.

CHAPTER 11

Money Matters and Legal Issues

Once you know the diagnosis is Alzheimer's, start planning immediately for a time when the person with AD can no longer make independent decisions. Coming to grips with the financial and legal consequences of a serious illness such as Alzheimer's is complicated and difficult. To ensure your loved one's care and comfort, it is essential that you talk with a lawyer about health and end-of-life wishes; how to manage your loved one's finances; and how to pay for long-term Alzheimer's care, which experts say costs many families as much as $200,000.

Essential Planning

Professionals encourage anyone recently diagnosed with a serious illness, especially one that is potentially debilitating, to examine and update their financial and health care arrangements as soon as possible. That means gathering and reviewing financial records, wills, trusts, and advance directives and perhaps putting new ones in place. Prompt financial and legal planning is particularly important with Alzheimer's because the disease gradually impairs the ability to reason and make decisions about how to manage money, assets, and health.

Laws governing health care and finance decisions are enormously complicated and vary from state to state, so you should probably consult a lawyer who can help you ensure that your loved one's wishes are carried out and your family's needs are addressed. An attorney can also advise you about how changes in a situation— for instance, a divorce, relocation, or death in the family—can influence legal documents and arrangements.

 Alert

> When possible, advance planning should take place soon after a diagnosis of early-stage AD, while the person can participate in discussions. People with early-stage AD are often capable of understanding many aspects and consequences of legal decision-making, according to the Alzheimer's Disease Education and Referral Center (ADEAR).

Your loved one's papers should all be in one place. Make sure you know where they are. An attorney who specializes in elder law can be particularly helpful in planning your finances and helping you learn how to conserve and spend financial assets while you are caring for a loved one.

Directives for Financial and Estate Management

Advance directives for financial and estate management must be created while the person with AD has the legal capacity to make decisions; in other words, while he is still capable of making them. If a court finds that a person with dementia is legally incompetent— incapable of making decisions about his medical care or property—the court can appoint a legal guardian (sometimes called a conservator) to make decisions about his custody and care. The person with dementia—or someone else involved in his care—can object to the guardianship, and the court may hold a hearing if that occurs. If there is no objection, a guardian is appointed.

You will need to create several documents. Each has its own function. Among legal documents that must be prepared are these:

❏ A will indicates how a person's assets and estate will be distributed upon death. The will may also specify arrangements for care of minors; creation of gifts or trusts; and funeral and/or burial arrangements.

❏ A durable power of attorney for finances authorizes an appointed person (agent) to manage and make decisions about the income and assets (property) of the person with dementia (principal). This decision-maker is responsible to act according to the instructions and in the best interests of the person who appointed her.

❏ A living trust provides instructions about the person's estate and appoints a trustee to hold title to property and funds for beneficiaries. The trustee follows these instructions after the person can no longer manage his affairs.

 Alert

A person with dementia maintains the right to make his own decisions—as long as he is competent—even if others disagree with his decisions. Power of attorney does not give an appointed person the authority to override the decision-making of the person with dementia.

Health Care Directives and Documents

Advance directives for health care and their related documents are almost always prepared while a person is legally able to execute them. These documents and their functions include the following:

❏ A durable power of attorney for health care designates an individual, sometimes called an agent or proxy, to make health care decisions for someone with AD if and when she can no longer do so. A health care proxy may be authorized to refuse or agree to treatments, change health care providers, remove a patient from an institution, and decide about making organ donations. If the patient's wishes aren't specified in a living will, a health care proxy may also be authorized to determine whether to begin or continue life support.

❑ A living will records a person's wishes for medical treatment near the end of life. A living will may specify the extent of life-sustaining treatment and major medical intervention. It often specifies the amount of discretion given to a health care proxy to make end-of-life decisions.

❑ A do not resuscitate (DNR) order, signed by a doctor and put in a person's medical chart, instructs health care professionals not to perform cardiopulmonary resuscitation if a person's heart stops or if she stops breathing.

Advance health care and financial planning can help people diagnosed with AD and their families confront tough questions about future treatment, caregiving, and legal arrangements. Although difficult issues may arise, advance planning can help all of you clarify wishes and make well-informed decisions in both the short term and long term.

Finding an Attorney

Consider consulting the National Academy of Elder Law Attorneys, a resource for information, education, referrals, and assistance to people dealing with the specialized legal needs of older people. The organization's website (*www.naela.org*) features education publications and videos on legal and financial concerns of people living with chronic illness.

You can do advance planning with documents downloaded from federal and state government websites. Contact the American

Bar Association, your nearby Area Agency on Aging (AAA) offices, and state legal aid associations if you can't afford legal help.

Covering the Costs of Alzheimer's Care

You may assume that private insurance, retiree benefits, and government programs such as Medicare will pay for long-term dementia care. Unfortunately, that is not always the case. People with AD and their families pay for many necessary services out of their own pockets.

Fact

Medicare beneficiaries age sixty-five and over spend close to one-quarter of their incomes on health care costs, according to the AARP. Nearly half of that money goes toward Medicare Part B premiums, private Medicare plans (such as HMOs), and private supplemental insurance purchased to cover gaps in Medicare coverage.

Medicare covers most hospital and other health care services for older people. Individuals and their families cover the cost of Medicare premiums, deductibles, copayments, and other health care expenses that are not covered by the federal insurance program.

Basic Expenses

The type and level of care a person with AD needs changes over time. The Alzheimer's Association advises that you anticipate paying for these and other needs:

- Ongoing medical treatment, diagnosis, and follow-up visits
- Treatment for other medical conditions
- Prescription drugs
- Personal care supplies
- Adult day services

- In-home care services
- Residential care services, including assisted living and nursing homes

The phrase *long-term care* describes a range of health and support services, including personal care and assistance with activities of daily living. Many family caregivers provide people with Alzheimer's all or much of this care free. As Alzheimer's progresses and a patient's needs increase, nearly all family caregivers find they have to supplement their own care with paid assistance, either at home or in an assisted living or nursing home facility.

Alert

The out-of-pocket cost of caring for an aging parent or spouse averages about $5,500 a year, according to a 2007 survey. On average, caregivers spend 10 percent of their household income to manage the extra expenses of providing "free" home-based care.

The cost of these services varies according to where you live, what kind of help you need, and how much of it you use. Very often, the services aren't covered by Medicare. The average costs of long-term care in the United States (as of 2008) are:

- ❏ $187/day for a semi-private room in a nursing home
- ❏ $209/day for a private room in a nursing home
- ❏ $3,008/month for care in an assisted living facility (for a one-bedroom unit)
- ❏ $29/hour for a home health aide
- ❏ $18/hour for homemaker services
- ❏ $59/day for care in an adult day health center care

Source: *U.S. Department of Health and Human Services National Clearinghouse for Long-term Care Information*

Fact

According to a 2005 Pew Research Center report, 10 million baby boomers are raising children or supporting an adult child while providing financial support to an aging parent. Balancing health care and living expenses for their parents with their children's college tuition has drained the financial resources of many baby boomers.

Understanding the costs, benefits, and long-term ramifications of dementia care is difficult under the best of circumstances. It can be extremely perplexing for people dealing with an AD diagnosis. Seek the advice of professional financial advisers who can help you find and tap into potential financial resources; learn about and take advantage of tax deductions; and avoid bad financial transactions and investment decisions that could deplete your finances.

Ways to Pay for Alzheimer's Care

Most people tap into several sources to help pay for dementia care. Those include:

❑ **Private and public insurance:** disability insurance from an employer-paid plan or personal policy, a group employee plan or retiree medical coverage, life insurance, long-term care insurance, and the government programs Medicare and Medigap.

❑ **Retirement benefits:** individual retirement accounts (IRAs) and employee-funded retirement plans, such as a 401(k), 403(b), and Keogh accounts.

❑ **Personal savings and assets:** cash, stocks, bonds, real estate, and personal property.

❑ **Government assistance:** veterans' benefits, social security disability income (SSDI) for workers under age sixty-five; supplemental security income (SSI), Medicaid, and tax credits and deductions.

❑ **Community support:** free or subsidized transportation, meal delivery, support groups, and respite care.

Fact

Some families turn life insurance policies into cash to help pay for AD care. Others use reverse mortgages. Consult the Alzheimer's Association's "Money Matters" brochure for more information. It's available online at *www.alz.org*.

To see if you may be eligible for a variety of governmental programs, check the National Council on Aging Benefits Checkup at *www.benefitscheckup.org*.

Sources of Assistance

* Medicare, a federal health insurance program for people age sixty-five or older and some with disabilities, generally covers all inpatient hospital care once you meet your deductible. Medicare also covers up to 80 percent of "reasonable and necessary" doctor's fees, some physical and mental therapies, medical items, and some of the costs of outpatient prescription drugs. The program also covers the cost of some home health care—including skilled nursing care and rehabilitation therapy—under certain conditions, for a limited time. Note that Medicare does not pay for long-term nursing home care. Most people purchase a supplement to Medicare coverage, such as Medigap.
* Medigap is a secondary insurance, sold by private health insurance brokers nationwide, that covers gaps in Medicare

coverage. It is regulated by federal and state laws that vary from state to state. The more expensive Medigap policies may cover additional items such as the deductibles on other insurance policies and out-of-pocket copayments. Medigap is meant to supplement Medicare. It does not cover anything Medicare won't pay for, including long-term care.

- Disability insurance provides income for a worker who can no longer work due to illness or injury. An employer-paid disability policy provides 60 to 70 percent of a person's gross income.

- Social security disability income is for workers younger than sixty-five who meet the Social Security Administration's definition of disability. To qualify, you will likely have to prove that the person with dementia is unable to work in any occupation, that the condition will last at least a year, or that it is expected to result in death.

- Supplemental security income guarantees a minimum monthly income for people who are age sixty-five or older. It also covers people under age sixty-five who are disabled or blind and those with very little income and few assets.

- Medicaid pays the costs of medical care for low-income people with few assets. It also covers long-term care for people who have used up most of their own money. Medicaid is the only federal program that will cover the long nursing home stays that most people with dementia require, but this program also requires beneficiaries to be poor to receive coverage.

Long-term care insurance typically pays for the costs of most long-term residential facilities, including nursing homes if you purchased a long-term care policy that covers Alzheimer's before you were diagnosed with symptoms of the disease. It's very unlikely you will be able to purchase long-term health insurance to cover the costs of the disease once Alzheimer's has already been diagnosed.

Tax Benefits for Caregivers

If a person with dementia is dependent under the tax rules, caregivers may be able to use their own workplace flexible spending account to cover the person's medical costs or dependent care expenses.

Federal Tax Deductions

If you are taking care of a chronically ill person—and if she is dependent according to state and federal tax rules—you may qualify for income tax deductions, according to the Alzheimer's Association. You qualify for federal income tax deductions only if you are caring for someone who has been certified chronically ill by a licensed health care practitioner within the previous twelve months. A professional clinician must prescribe your services.

L. Essential

If you are caring for someone with AD, keep receipts and records of everything you spend on services and care, from receipts for heating pads to home repair to physical therapy. Be sure, too, to save copies of all medical assessments, prescriptions, certifications, and plans of care.

Deductible expenses may include personal care items, such as disposable briefs and special foods; home improvements, such as grab bars; in-home care, such as physical or occupational therapy; nursing services; and some long-term residential care.

State Taxes

Most states and the District of Columbia provide some assistance with the costs of Alzheimer's care that aren't covered by insurance plans. (State tax credits and deductions vary by state.)

Some states provide a caregiver tax credit to help cover the expense of caring for a chronically ill person in your home. Most states require that the caregiver live with the disabled person for at least six months of the year. Each state has different qualifying expenses and different credit amounts. Always consult a competent tax professional for advice about understanding and applying tax laws in your situation and your state. If your loved one is a qualifying dependent—a person of any age who lives with you and is physically or mentally incapable of caring for herself—and you pay someone to care for her so you can work, you may qualify for your state's child and dependent care credit.

Many states allow for a deduction of medical expenses for long-term care services if the chronically ill person is certified by a physician and prescribed a plan of care. Many states allow you to claim a credit or deduction for long-term care insurance premiums. In most states, the insurance policy must qualify for the benefit under federal law or be authorized by the state.

CHAPTER 12

Treating Alzheimer's Symptoms

Medications can't halt or cure Alzheimer's, but some drugs can treat certain symptoms of AD. The U.S. Food and Drug Administration (FDA) has approved five prescription medicines that target memory loss and other cognitive symptoms of dementia. Other FDA-approved medications treat psychological symptoms, such as depression, and behavioral problems, such as anger and aggression, in people with AD. While none of these drugs will stop or reverse the progression of Alzheimer's, they may ease symptoms and provide comfort.

Drugs That Treat Cognitive Symptoms

The FDA has approved five drugs to treat memory loss and other cognitive symptoms of dementia. All of these drugs help influence brain chemical activity. Four of the drugs—donepezil (Aricept), galantamine (Razadyne, formerly Reminyl), rivastigmine (Exelon), and tacrine (Cognex)—are known as cholinesterase inhibitors. The fifth, memantine (Namenda), belongs to a class of medications known as NMDA receptor antagonists.

Cholinesterase Inhibitors
Cholinesterase inhibitors are drugs that block the activity of an enzyme in the brain called cholinesterase, which breaks apart the

neurotransmitter acetylcholine, a chemical messenger involved in memory, learning, and judgment. Cholinesterase inhibitors reduce the action of cholinesterase, thereby making more acetylcholine available to nerve cells in the brain.

Fact

Doctors' opinions vary considerably about whether to prescribe medications for Alzheimer's symptoms before trying nondrug strategies like stress reduction or behavior modification. Most medications work best in combination with interventions such as psychotherapy and stress reduction. .

Experts agree that these medications are only moderately successful in treating cognitive symptoms of AD. In general, they delay the worsening of AD symptoms for six to twelve months in approximately half of the people who take them. Some patients' symptoms improve dramatically, but as many as half experience no noticeable improvement. The four cholinesterase inhibitors approved to treat different stages of AD differ from one another slightly:

- **Donepezil** (Aricept), the most frequently prescribed cholinesterase inhibitor, prevents the breakdown of acetylcholine in the brain. It accounts for approximately 70 percent of all prescriptions written for cholinesterase inhibitors, in part because it is approved to treat mild, moderate, and severe stages of Alzheimer's disease.
- **Rivastigmine** (Exelon) prevents the breakdown of both acetylcholine and a similar chemical, butyrylcholine, in the brain. It is approved to treat mild to moderate Alzheimer's.

- **Galantamine** (Razadyne), formerly known as Reminyl, prevents the breakdown of acetylcholine. It also stimulates nicotine receptors to release more acetylcholine in the brain. It is approved to treat mild to moderate Alzheimer's.
- **Tacrine** (Cognex), the first cholinesterase inhibitor, was approved in 1993 but is rarely prescribed today because of its side effects, which include possible liver damage.

None of these drugs has proven more clinically effective than another, according to the American Academy of Family Physicians. And there is no evidence that combining two or three of them would improve their results, doctors say. Combining the drugs appears to cause more side effects.

Alert

Do not stop taking a drug without consulting your doctor or another medical professional. Many AD patients are extremely sensitive to the effects of medications, but discontinuing a drug abruptly can cause serious physical and mental problems. Withdrawing from drugs prescribed to treat cognitive difficulties may cause symptoms to worsen suddenly and severely.

Some patients have shown improvement taking doses higher than those regularly recommended for each drug. But higher-than-recommended doses are also likely to cause more side effects.

Each cholinesterase inhibitor varies slightly from the others in its chemical makeup, and one drug may work better for a particular patient than it does another. Check with your doctor if you experience any of the most common side effects to see if a similar medication might work for you. Many side effects can be reduced or avoided altogether by taking a drug in different doses or at different times of day.

Namenda (Memantine)

Namenda was widely used in Europe for more than twenty years before it was approved to treat moderate and severe Alzheimer's in the United States in 2003. Namenda regulates the activity of glutamate, another messenger chemical involved in learning and memory. It is thought to be equally as effective as cholinesterase inhibitors in temporarily delaying worsening of symptoms in some people.

Question

What are the side effects of cholinesterase inhibitors?
Most patients can tolerate cholinesterase inhibitors, which cause relatively few side effects in most patients. Nausea, vomiting, loss of appetite, and increased frequency of bowel movements are the most frequently reported side effects.

Because Namenda works differently than cholinesterase inhibitors in the brain, it may be prescribed in combination with one of those drugs, according to the National Institute on Aging. Some doctors report that people given Aricept with Namenda do better than those taking Aricept alone.

DRUGS THAT TREAT ALZHEIMER'S DISEASE

Drug name	Approved for	Common Side Effects
Donepezil (Aricept)	mild, moderate, and severe AD	nausea, diarrhea, vomiting
Galantamine (Razadyne)	mild to moderate AD	nausea, vomiting, diarrhea, weight loss
Rivastigmine (Exelon)	mild to moderate AD	nausea, vomiting, weight loss, upset stomach, muscle weakness
Memantine (Namenda)	mild to moderate AD	dizziness, headache, constipation, confusion

Source: *U.S. Department of Health and Human Services*

Treating Psychological Problems

Depression and anxiety are extremely common among people with Alzheimer's, and doctors frequently prescribe medication to treat symptoms of those conditions. Research shows, however, that drug therapy for psychological problems usually works best when it is combined with nondrug treatments such as counseling, stress reduction, and behavior modification.

Treating Depression

Most anti-depressant drugs currently prescribed are tricyclic antidepressants or selective serotonin reuptake inhibitors (SSRIs).

First prescribed in the 1950s, tricyclics were the preferred pharmacological approach to treating depression for many years, and the drugs are still considered effective. All are available as generics. But tricyclics may take weeks to show their effects and can cause irritating side effects—weight gain and dry mouth as well as more serious side effects such as irregular heartbeat and impaired memory in some patients.

Most doctors today prefer SSRIs, a newer generation of drugs designed to increase levels of serotonin—a neurotransmitter that influences mood, emotion, appetite, and sleep—in the brain. SSRIs, believed to be generally safe and effective in treating depression in older adults and people with dementia, seem to cause relatively few side effects in most people. They can, however, increase anxiety and agitation in people who already suffer those symptoms.

Medications that are frequently prescribed for AD patients suffering depression, apathy, and irritability include the following:

- citalopram (Celexa)
- fluoxetine (Prozac)
- paroxetine (Paxil)

- sertraline (Zoloft)
- trazodone (Desyrel)

Calming Anxiety

If anxiety interferes with an AD patient's overall ability to function (if, for example, nervousness discourages him from leaving the house), the doctor may prescribe one among a family of drugs known as benzodiazepines. lorazepam (Ativan), oxazepam (Serax), buspirone (Buspar) and zolpidem (Ambien) are the most popular of these drugs.

Question

Should doctors prescribe drugs currently available to treat Alzheimer's, even though the benefits are modest?
The American College of Physicians and the American Academy of Family Physicians refused to make blanket recommendations on the drugs in 2008, when they issued guidelines to clinicians. The organization urged doctors to decide whether to prescribe drugs on a case-by-case basis, taking into consideration the patient's overall health profile, her tolerance of side effects, the ease of taking the medication, and its cost.

Benzodiazepines are considered effective sedatives, and they can help combat agitation and sleeplessness—common complaints of AD patients. But they are addicting and their effectiveness tends to decrease the longer a patient takes them. Experts advise using them with caution for short intervals.

Treating Sleeplessness

Many physicians are reluctant to prescribe sleep aids for older adults with dementia because such patients are particularly susceptible to the serious side effects those medications can cause, such as agitation, balance problems, and incontinence. Physicians also urge dementia patients to avoid over-the-counter sleep remedies. The active ingredient in many medicines, the antihistamine diphenhydramine (Benadryl), is particularly problematic for people with AD because it can slow brain cell messenger chemicals that are already impeded by Alzheimer's.

 Alert

People with Alzheimer's disease should avoid over-the-counter sleep aids containing diphenhydramine, including Compoz, Nytol, Sominex, and Unisom, according to the national Alzheimer's Association. Keep in mind that diphenhydramine is also an ingredient in many nighttime versions of popular pain relievers and cold and sinus remedies.

Effective treatment of one symptom sometimes helps relieve others. Anti-anxiety medications and some antidepressants such as trazodone (Desyrel) make some people sleepy and may be helpful in treating insomnia in AD patients.

Treating Behavioral Problems

Antipsychotic medications, also known as neuroleptics, are used to quell some of the more disruptive and disturbing symptoms of mid- to late-stage Alzheimer's, including hallucinations, delusions, aggression, agitation, hostility, and uncooperativeness.

The drugs are extremely potent and are associated with serious side effects such as weight gains of thirty pounds or more in many people. The Alzheimer's Association warns that they should be used with extreme caution in people with dementia, who are susceptible to serious side effects, including stroke and an increased risk of death from antipsychotic medications.

No drug is FDA-approved to treat behavioral and psychiatric dementia symptoms. Those used most often—aripiprazole (Abilify), clozapine (Clozaril), haloperidol (Haldol), olanzapine (Zyprexa), quetiapine (Seroquel), risperidone (Risperdal), and ziprasidone (Geodon)—are prescribed for symptoms other than those for which they were tested and approved.

📋 Fact

Some antipsychotics worsen the symptoms they are prescribed to treat. Alzheimer's specialists urge doctors to prescribe drugs for behavioral problems only to target specific symptoms. That way, their effectiveness can be monitored and evaluated in deciding whether to increase, decrease, or discontinue the drug.

If you and your doctor are considering using antipsychotic drugs to treat AD symptoms, you should ask the following questions:

- ❏ What problem does this drug treat, and how effective is it?
- ❏ What improvements might we expect?
- ❏ How will this medication interact—or interfere with—treatments for other conditions?
- ❏ What are the most common side effects? Which should we watch for?
- ❏ How long do you expect it will take for the drug to show benefits?
- ❏ How will you evaluate the drug's effectiveness?
- ❏ How will you evaluate whether and when to stop using the drug?

A comprehensive study published in 2006 showed that these medications may be less effective than previously thought for use in treating symptoms of dementia. That year, the FDA issued a black-box warning about a slight—but statistically significant—increased risk of death in people with dementia who are taking antipsychotic medications. An FDA review of seventeen studies of off-label use of antipsychotics in treating dementia suggested that while certain antipsychotics are useful in reducing aggression and/or psychosis, they should not be used routinely with dementia patients, unless a patient is in severe distress and will not respond to other treatments.

AD experts and federal health officials advise using antipsychotics only when a patient's symptoms are caused by mania or psychosis, endanger the patient or other people, or make it extremely difficult to provide necessary care. Antipsychotic medications should never be used to sedate or restrain someone with dementia. In all cases, doctors should prescribe the lowest effective dosage for the least amount of time possible.

Helpful Tips for Monitoring Medications

Many people with AD are older, and many older people take several medications at once. Here are some suggestions, adapted from the Mayo Clinic, to help you keep track of daily medication needs:

❑ Write and regularly update a list of medications, dosages, and the time of day all vitamins and pills should be taken. Post it inside a kitchen cupboard door.

❑ Keep a list of common side effects and other information about medication.

❑ Use a weekly pillbox, available at any pharmacy, to sort medications and keep track of whether they've been taken. Label the pillboxes (Susie, 8 A.M.; Susie, lunchtime).

❑ Check the pillbox to be sure the pills have been taken.

❑ Use alarms and reminders such as phone calls to help keep the patient on schedule.

❑ Post your doctor's emergency phone number and the number of a local poison control center near all phones in case of accidental overdose.

In addition, it's helpful to keep the following precautions in mind when you consider prescription drugs:

❑ Be sure you take medications under the supervision of a physician who is experienced in treating and monitoring patients who take AD drugs.

❑ Understand the specific symptoms the medication is prescribed to treat; for example, confusion or memory problems.

❑ Ask why the doctor prescribed this particular medication rather than another.

❑ Ask how effective the doctor expects the drug will be in treating symptoms and how she will measure its effectiveness.

❑ Be sure the doctor knows about all prescription medications, herbal supplements, or over-the-counter medications the patient is taking. Some over-the-counter allergy medications such as Benadryl and herbal supplements such as St. John's wort may interfere with AD medications.

❑ Ask the doctor to review and adjust medications if necessary.

❑ Start by taking the lowest effective dose of any drug and increase it gradually if necessary.

❑ Do not stop taking the drugs if you don't feel noticeable improvement in your symptoms.

❑ Call a health care professional immediately if the drug causes severe side effects. Continuing to take the medication could cause serious health issues.

Paying for Medications

The price of most AD drugs is high—$148 to $195 a month, according to Consumer Reports—and you may worry about whether you can afford your prescription medications. Fortunately, you may be eligible to receive help paying for the drugs your doctor recommends.

Your doctor or research center may give you free samples of drugs you take, and nearly all pharmaceutical manufacturers have patient-assistance programs that provide or point you to sources of free or low-cost medication. Visit their websites.

BenefitsCheckUp

You may want to begin by visiting the BenefitsCheckUp website (*www.benefitscheckup.org*), a service of the National Council on Aging (NCOA), which can help you determine what drug programs you may be eligible for and provide detailed instructions on how to enroll.

Plan D Medicare Coverage

All Medicare beneficiaries are eligible for prescription drug coverage. For details about drug benefits for people with AD, visit the Medicare Prescription Drug Plan finder on the agency website, *www.medicare.gov.*

Partnership for Prescription Assistance

This one-stop online information source offers a single point of access to more than 475 public and private patient assistance programs, including more than 150 programs offered by pharmaceutical companies. Call 888-477-2669 or visit *www.pparx.org* to see which programs you or a loved one may be eligible for. You will have to answer questions or fill out an online application.

CHAPTER 13

Questions and Answers about Clinical Trials

Clinical trials are carefully designed, controlled investigations that determine whether a promising treatment is safe and effective for human use. They are important in finding new, reliable ways to treat Alzheimer's. A good clinical trial can allow you to take an active role in your own health care as you contribute to medical research. Medications and techniques that are not yet approved for widespread use may be your best option for treatment, but there are risks to consider, too.

What Is a Clinical Trial?

Experimental drugs and treatments are tested and evaluated in four phases of study, or trials. These phases are explained in detail later in this chapter. In preclinical studies, scientists gather information and evidence from laboratory research, animal testing, and human observational trials indicating that a treatment shows promise and that it would provide a benefit that current medications don't.

In clinical trials, volunteer subjects work with a research team of doctors, nurses, and other health professionals at private research facilities, teaching hospitals, AD research centers, or doctors' offices. Researchers and volunteers follow a protocol—a study plan that determines who may participate in the trial (people with early-stage AD or those already taking medication, for example); the schedule of tests, treatments, and procedures involved; and the length of the study. The protocol is designed to assure the health and well-being of participants as it answers questions about the treatment.

Most clinical trials randomly assign participants to a study group. One group, the test or control group, is given the experimental drug or treatment. Other groups may receive a different drug or a placebo, an inactive substance that looks like the study drug. Only by comparing the groups can researchers be sure that changes among patients in the test group are caused by the treatment, not something else.

What Happens During a Clinical Trial?

The clinical trial process depends on the kind of trial being conducted. All trials follow a protocol, and in all trials a clinical team checks your health at the beginning of the trial, gives you specific instructions for participating, monitors your progress during the trial, and stays in touch after the trial is completed, according to the National Institutes of Health. Some clinical trials involve more tests and doctor visits than do others. There also are other differences among the types of clinical trials:

- Treatment trials test experimental treatments, new drug combinations, and approaches to medical interventions such as surgery or radiation therapy. Some of these trials test the safety of brand new treatments, while others assess whether a drug already approved by the FDA for one purpose is useful for other purposes. (For example, several treatment trials for Alzheimer's have focused on anti-inflammatory agents, already approved to treat arthritis, which show some promise in treating people with AD.)
- Prevention trials research better ways to stave off a disease among those who have never had it, or to keep it from returning in patients who have. These trials focus not only on medi-

cines and vaccines, but on vitamins, minerals, and lifestyle changes that fall within the realm of complementary care.

- Diagnostic trials look for better tests and procedures for diagnosing a disease or condition.
- Screening trials look for improved ways of detecting a disease or health condition.
- Quality of life trials, also known as supportive care trials, explore ways of improving comfort and quality of life for people with chronic illness and their caregivers.

Why Volunteer for a Clinical Trial?

Anyone considering volunteering for a study should understand the rewards and risks involved before making a decision.

Benefits

Patients who participate in clinical trials frequently have access to promising new treatments before they are widely available. They receive regular, quality care during the course of the study and generally have access to the health professionals on the study team and staff. The quality of care provided during clinical studies, which are generally conducted at top-notch medical centers, tends to be quite high.

Drawbacks

Clinical trials generally don't have miraculous results, warn federal health experts at ADEAR. The test drug or treatment may relieve a symptom, delay the severity of symptoms, or reduce your risk of death. On the other hand, the treatment may not help you. It might cause side effects. You should also consider whether the test protocol requires too large an investment of your time, travel, or money.

Some patients and families have a hard time with the uncertainties of clinical trials. They dislike not knowing which study group they're in and whether they're taking a drug or placebo.

Some participants grow impatient because it can take a long time to learn whether the trial was successful or not.

Essential

Research shows that people who are involved in studies tend to do somewhat better than people in a similar stage of their disease who are not enrolled—regardless of whether the experimental treatment works, says the Alzheimer's Association.

Learn as much as you can about clinical trials in general before you think of volunteering. Get detailed information about a study before you decide to participate in it.

Inform yourself

Here are some questions you may want to ask the health care study team:

❏ What is the purpose of the study? What do you hope to learn?
❏ Who is going to be in the study?
❏ Why is this treatment being tested? Why do researchers think it may be effective? Has it been tested before?
❏ What kinds of tests and experimental treatments are involved?
❏ What are the possible risks, side effects, and benefits to me in the study?
❏ How much involvement will it require?
❏ How long will the trial last?
❏ Who will pay for the experimental treatment?
❏ Will I be reimbursed for certain expenses, like travel?

Source: *ClinicalTrials.gov*

Who Can Participate in Clinical Trials?

All clinical trial protocols include inclusion/exclusion criteria: strict rules about who can and can't participate. The criteria are usually based on age, gender, the stage of your disease, previous treatment history, and other medical conditions, and you must fit the inclusion criteria to qualify for the study.

⌴ Essential

If you are considering participating in a clinical study, you and your family have a right to be thoroughly informed about the nature of the study and any potential risks. You have a right to clear, detailed answers to your questions—and to expect that study staff will repeat and explain information so you understand it.

Inclusion and exclusion criteria are not used to accept or reject you personally, but to ensure that researchers can answer the questions the trial is designed to study. Some seek participants with illnesses or conditions to be studied in the clinical trial, while others need healthy participants. Some want women; others need men. One trial might test AD treatments in people with a family history of the disease.

How Safe Are Clinical Trials?

All biomedical research involving people that is conducted in the United States must be approved and monitored by an institutional review board (IRB). This independent committee, which is made up of physicians, statisticians, community advocates, and others, approves, monitors, and reviews biomedical and behavioral research involving human subjects and is charged with protecting their rights and welfare. Most clinical trials are federally regulated and adhere to government-mandated medical and ethical practices.

As a clinical trial progresses, researchers report the results of the trial at scientific meetings, to medical journals, and to various government agencies, which assures additional transparency of the study. Individual participants' names will remain secret and will not be mentioned in these reports.

Avoiding Human Error

People sometimes feel better—and some even perform better on medical tests—if they think a treatment is helping them. And doctors sometimes convince themselves that a certain treatment is helping a patient because the physician really wants the patient to get better.

Clinical trials are designed to screen out these normal, unscientific human biases, which can skew results of scientific tests. That is why they follow these procedures:

- Most Phase II and Phase III clinical trials are randomized studies, in which participants are randomly assigned to one treatment or another.
- Most trials are placebo-controlled. Participants are selected at random, usually by computer, to receive the experimental treatment or a placebo that looks and tastes like a drug but has no effect.
- Clinical trials are blind or double-blind. In blind studies, subjects don't know which treatment they receive. In double-blind studies, neither the subjects nor the study staff know which patients are taking a drug and which are getting the placebo.

How Are Clinical Trials Organized?

Drugs and procedures don't advance to clinical trials unless they show some significant promise of improving or preventing a condition and researchers think their rewards outweigh their risks. Clinical trials involve human subjects, and they are carefully designed to assure effectiveness and safety.

Phase I Trials

In the first phase of human testing, researchers test an experimental drug or treatment in a small number of volunteers (fewer than 100). They study safety, risks, and side effects. Phase I trials generally last only a few months.

 Fact

Researchers often submit data to the U.S. Food and Drug Administration (FDA) for review and approval during Phase III trials. Most drugs undergo two successful Phase III trials before the FDA approves them, according to health and safety authorities at the National Institutes of Health.

Phase II Trials

If an experimental drug or treatment fulfills criteria in Phase I, it moves to Phase II trials, which typically enroll a few hundred volunteers. The treatment is tested for safety and efficacy among a larger group of people (typically between 100 and 300) over longer periods of time.

Phase III Trials

Drugs and treatments that pass muster in the earlier trials are tested in large groups of hundreds or thousands of patients, depending on what is being studied. Phase III trials are designed to definitively evaluate the effectiveness of a drug or treatment, and to compare it with the best current treatments and practices.

Phase IV Trials

Phase IV trials, also known as post-marketing surveillance trials, monitor the safety, risks, benefits, and competitive advantages of an FDA-approved drug that is already on the market.

Giving Your Consent

If you are interested in and accepted to a study, you will be asked to sign an informed consent, which outlines everything you need to know about the trial and the rules and regulations that protect you. Laws and regulations regarding informed consent differ across states and research institutions, but most are modeled after the informed consent policies of the federal government.

Informed Consent

Federal law requires that the following information be provided to each subject:

1. A statement that the study involves research, an explanation of the purposes of the research, how long you are expected to participate, and what procedures are to be followed. Any experimental procedures must be identified.
2. A description of any reasonably foreseeable risks or discomforts you might experience.
3. A description of any benefits to you or to others that might reasonably be expected from the research.
4. A disclosure of appropriate alternative procedures or courses of treatment, if any, that might be advantageous to you.
5. A statement describing the extent to which records identifying you will be kept confidential, and a note that the FDA may inspect the records.
6. If the research involves more than minimal risk, the consent form should provide details about whether patients

will be compensated and whether any medical treatments are available should injury occur. Those details should describe what compensations and treatments consist of, or where further information may be obtained.

7. Names and numbers of authorities the patients can call with questions about the research study and research subjects' rights, and in the event of a research-related injury.

8. A statement that participation is voluntary, that refusal to participate will involve no penalty or loss of benefits to which you are otherwise entitled, and that you may discontinue participation at any time without penalty or loss of benefits to which you are otherwise entitled.

Fact

The U.S. National Institutes of Health offers comprehensive, up-to-date information on all clinical trials currently underway in the United States at *www.clinicaltrials.gov* and through the Alzheimer's Disease Education and Referral Center (ADEAR) Clinical Trials Database at *www.alzheimers.org/clinicaltrials*. The Alzheimer's Association (*www. alz.org*) is also an excellent source of information for those who are considering participating in clinical trials.

Depending on the study protocol, the informed consent may also include warnings that a particular treatment or procedure may pose unforeseeable risks and provide details of additional costs you may incur while participating in research. For more details on informed consent, visit the FDA's website at *www.fda.gov*.

What Is Usually Involved?

Once you are accepted into a study, you will have an introductory visit with the study staff. Typically, you will undergo a thorough physical exam as well as extensive cognitive and physical testing during this visit. If you're testing a drug or treatment, you will receive it during this visit. You will be asked to follow a strict medication or treatment protocol, or instructions, and to keep detailed records of your symptoms.

Once the trial is under way, you will make periodic visits to the clinic or research center for physical and cognitive exams, to give blood and urine samples, and to talk with study staff. The information gathered during these visits helps researchers measure the effects of the treatment, monitor your progress, and answer questions from you and your caregiver.

What to Expect During a Clinical Trial

You may experience side effects, which are unwanted reactions to a drug or treatment. Common adverse effects include headache, nausea, hair loss, skin irritation, sleepiness, or excitability. Experimental treatments are evaluated for both short- and long-term side effects.

You can continue to see your regular doctors and caregivers during the trial. Clinicians involved in most studies will treat you for specific, short-term illnesses or conditions, but they are not primary health care providers. You can leave a clinical trial at any time. If you withdraw from a trial, you should let the research team know you are leaving and tell them why.

You Can Make a Difference!

At any given time, more than 150 clinical studies are recruiting participants with and without Alzheimer's disease, related diseases, or memory loss to help test exciting new approaches.

Clinical studies are the engine that drives medical progress, made up of human energy. Scientists work continually to find better ways to treat diseases. Improved treatments can never become a reality without testing in human volunteers.

CHAPTER 14

Changing Behavior

P eople in the middle or moderate stages of Alzheimer's disease lose their memory functioning, independence, and sense of self. Communicating is difficult, because they have trouble following what's said to them and making themselves clear. Some become restless and agitated. Others are fearful and suspicious. Some swear, scream, throw things, and even hit, kick, or bite. You can't control the disease that causes this behavior, but you may be able to soothe or calm some of its effects.

Behavior Basics

Behavior is a response to what is happening inside and around you. If you don't feel well or you're overtired, you probably don't think as clearly as you usually do. You may get disoriented, feel things are out of your control, and get frustrated or angry. Those are normal human responses that usually go away when you feel better. People with dementia, however, don't feel better. They become more tired and confused and less able to care for themselves.

There is no question that it's difficult to deal with hostile, uncooperative, and difficult behavior in someone with AD, particularly if you've been working hard to provide the best care and comfort you can. Try to remember that the behavior isn't stubbornness or mean-spiritedness. It's a response to a devastating illness.

Alzheimer's progresses steadily, but it affects the brain unevenly. That is why your father may recall details of his wedding day but forgets celebrating his fortieth wedding anniversary last summer, even though you showed him a video of the event last night. It's the reason your mother persists in unloading dirty dishes from your dishwasher and putting them away.

Essential

Alzheimer's destroys the brain's ability to learn from mistakes. Do not argue, threaten, or punish someone for behavior she can't control and may not recall later. The behavior you find frustrating may be a response to her basic human need to be busy and productive. Try to find a task for her, like folding laundry, that helps satisfy that need.

These relatively mild symptoms occur because AD damages the brain's ability to remember, learn, and reason. She doesn't remember emptying the dishwasher yesterday, or your asking her not to do it. She can't learn from her mistake because dementia afflicts her once sound judgment. She's confused and disoriented, so she can't tell that the dishes are dirty. All she knows is that they belong in the cupboard.

Behavior Responses

When someone with dementia bursts into tears or makes an angry accusation, it doesn't occur in a vacuum. Someone may have said something that upset her. She might be bothered by activity in the house, loud noises, or glaring light. Her stomach might be upset. She may not have slept well. All behavior is triggered. One way caregivers can change behavior is to change the pattern that leads to that behavior.

By identifying causes and patterns of disturbing behavior, you can modify the environment (by decreasing noise, for example) and the way you approach a confused person. Sometimes, simplifying a situation or decision can work wonders. For example, if a loved one becomes combative when trying to decide what to eat or wear, you can limit the choices available. Rather than suggesting, "Why don't you get dressed?" lay out clothing and say, "Why don't you put these clothes on?"

Alert

Sometimes it may be difficult to differentiate between the illness and the person you love. Learn to recognize the AD symptoms that contribute to her state of discomfort. Make an effort to understand what may have caused her distress and aggravated those symptoms.

If you're angry, upset, or bewildered by a loved one, take a breath, and HALT. Ask yourself if one of you is Hungry, Angry, Lonely, or Tired. If so, do what you can to change that situation.

Take Away the Triggers

People with brain diseases often become extremely upset, angry, or moody in certain situations. Going to a restaurant, spending the weekend at a relative's house, or being in a crowded room may feel so overwhelming and scary to someone that she overreacts to losing sight of you in a crowd, or being asked a question she doesn't understand. She may get angry or nasty, or burst into tears. She may train those emotions on you, the person trying to help.

To avoid these responses, it's important to recognize that these behaviors aren't stubbornness or nastiness, but a response to frustrating feelings the person can't help. Remember, too, that you actually have more control than she does, according to Johns Hopkins University dementia expert Peter V. Rabins, MD.

The best way to manage catastrophic reactions is to avoid things that upset the person you care for. Everyone responds differently, but certain situations trigger extreme reactions, sometimes called catastrophic responses, in many people. Among them are:

- Situations in which she has to think about and accomplish several tasks at once (such as bathing)
- Situations in which she is trying to do relatively simple things she can no longer manage on her own (putting away laundry or calling friends)
- Being cared for by someone who is rushed or rude
- Feeling inadequate because she can't follow a conversation or understand a doctor's questions
- Not understanding what she's asked to do
- Feeling tired
- Feeling frustrated
- Being treated like a child

MANAGING BEHAVIOR ISSUES

Valerie knew she needed help and support—and more than a weekly break from the demands of caring for her feeble, increasingly cranky mother.

But every caregiving book or website she looked at made her feel like she would never be able to provide consistent, loving care for her mother. She even avoided a caregiver help and support group at the local Y, she says, because she was "sure everyone was more patient and creative and loving than I can be on winter days when I'm stuck in the house with my mother.

"You don't get a lot of help and support in this job, but the expectations are really high," she points out. "You have a very sick person to take care of. You have to be a kid, a pal, a nurse, and whoever she thinks you are on the days she doesn't recognize you. You have to be really slow and quiet and patient, and really high-energy to get through some real hard days."

Valerie and her mother did not have a perfect relationship, she says. "I was a rebellious teenager, into my early twenties, really, and she was going through her own problems while dealing with mine, so we had some tough times. We've gotten along a lot better since then, and I was glad in a lot of ways to be able to take time off from work to take care of her.

"But when she's cranky and messy and she doesn't want to do anything, I get exasperated. I get hurt when she thinks I'm one of my sisters—and I think she wishes I was one of my sisters. And I get mad. Then I feel bad because I'm mad at this helpless little old person.

"I try not to be so hard on myself and remember the big picture. There are good moments and bad in all relationships, and overall, we're there for each other, so it's good. Hard, but good."

Agitation

Agitation describes a range of behaviors that are common among people with dementia, from irritability and insomnia to verbal outbursts or physical aggression. Mild agitation (irritation) often comes and goes in the early stages of AD, then grows more frequent and disruptive along with other symptoms. Occasional irritability can turn into frequent anger and then hostility.

Physical, environmental, or emotional triggers can set off agitation. It occurs most frequently, according to AD experts, when a person with dementia feels she is being forced to give up control—over what she eats, the clothes she wears, where she lives, or who is taking care of her.

Acknowledge a confused person's anger over losing control of her life. Tell her you understand her frustration. ("It's maddening, isn't it?") Other suggestions for soothing agitation:

- Try to cut down her caffeine, sugar, and junk food intake.
- Reduce noise, clutter, or activity.

- Make sure familiar, reassuring objects, such as furniture and photographs, surround her.
- Pat her hand. Rub her neck. Put on soothing music.
- Speak in a reassuring voice. Do not try to restrain the person during a period of agitation.
- Keep dangerous objects out of reach.

Keep in mind that confronting a confused person may increase her anxiety.

Repetition and Shadowing

People with dementia frequently repeat a single word, sentence, or question. They may repeat a gesture, such as brushing lint from a shirtsleeve or crumbling a tissue, over and over. This type of behavior is usually harmless for the person with dementia, but it can be annoying and stressful for others.

Essential

Be sensitive to how distressing it is for a mature adult to know she is losing the ability to do simple things she has always done for herself and others. Try to convey that you are helping her with basic tasks, not taking away more of her independence and dignity. Allow her to do as much for herself as possible.

Try to determine what may be triggering repetitive behavior: Is she asking when Jane is coming home because she's bored? Nervous? Afraid of being alone? Or is she fussing with clothing because she's uncomfortable or needs to use the bathroom?

It may make things easier if you don't discuss plans with a confused person until right before an event. If she's anticipating something (a meal or her son's arrival), you might be able to quell anxiety and uncertainty by putting a sign on the kitchen table announcing "Dinner at 6" or "David due home at 5" to remove anxiety and uncertainty.

Shadowing

People with dementia sometimes mimic whatever you are doing. They follow you around, talk incessantly, or interrupt what you are saying. This behavior often occurs late in the day and can be irritating for exhausted caregivers.

▤ Fact

> It is pointless to remind a person who asks a single question over and over that you've answered it six times. People with AD can't remember what they've asked or what you told them. Try distracting her with a snack or activity. Ignore the question for a while. Reassure her both in words and with touch.

Again, try to understand why she is following you. Comfort her with verbal and physical reassurance. Distract. Redirect. Try an activity or give her a task that makes her feel useful.

Suspicion and Paranoia

If someone you care for suddenly grows jealous or suspicious, sees things no one else does, or accuses you of something you haven't done, you will probably feel unsettled, hurt, or angry. Remember that whatever she is experiencing is very real to her. There is no point in arguing or disagreeing with someone who perceives something that isn't real. The best thing you can do is reassure her, perhaps helping her search for the source of her anxiety.

Help her look for things she thinks someone has taken. Try to find her favorite hiding places for storing objects she later reports as lost. Also, stock up on replacements for commonly lost items, such as wallets and hats.

Nonverbal reassurances like a gentle touch or hug can go a long way in comforting someone who is out of sorts because of dementia symptoms. Respond to the feeling behind the accusation and then reassure the person. You might try saying, "I see this frightens you; stay with me, I won't let anything happen to you."

Seeing Things

If your loved one sees or hears things no one else does and doesn't seem bothered by it, you shouldn't worry. If the pattern continues, speak with a doctor. Seeing shadows and patterns on a wall or reflections on a TV screen or in a mirror often triggers hallucinations in people with dementia. Sometimes a person with dementia may think she's heard something—children playing outdoors, for instance—or smelled something, like smoke from a barbecue grill, that may also make her think she's seen something that isn't there.

Redirect her attention to what you are saying. Try phrasing your responses like, "I see why you think that was a bat. It's a shadow."

⌶, Essential

If your loved one grows suspicious, be sure to explain to other family members, caregivers, and home helpers that her accusations are a part of her illness. This is particularly important with people who don't know her well, or with children and teenagers, who might not understand.

Your loved one is losing her ability to recognize faces and distinguish time and place. So if a grandson she hasn't seen in a while drops by to visit, she may mistake him for a stranger, either when he's there or later, when she's feeling anxious about something else. Or she might think he's the handyman she's been expecting and wonder why he's sitting down to chat, rather than fixing her sink.

Sundowning and Sleeplessness

Some people's AD symptoms seem to grow worse in the late afternoon or evening. They become particularly agitated and have trouble going to bed and staying asleep. Experts believe this behavior, commonly called sundowning, is caused by a combination of exhaustion and changes in the person's biological clock that confuse day and night.

Try to increase her activity during the daytime. Discourage napping. Watch out for foods that can increase insomnia, particularly in someone sensitive to it. Plan smaller meals throughout the day, including a light meal, such as half a sandwich, before bedtime.

Plan the day so afternoon and evening hours are quiet and calm but not boring or empty. Quiet, structured activity helps.

Fact

Delusions and hallucinations are psychotic symptoms. Delusions are unfounded but deeply felt ideas that often involve suspicion, paranoid thoughts, or inflated notions of self-importance. Delusions can also grow out of illness or hopelessness. Hallucinations are abnormal perceptions that involve one or more of the five senses (hearing, vision, touch, smell, and taste).

Turning on lights well before sunset and closing the curtains at dusk will minimize shadows and may help diminish confusion, dementia experts advise. Makes sure there are nightlights in the person's room, hallway, and bathroom.

Also be sure the house is safe. Block off stairs with gates, lock the kitchen door, and put away dangerous items. If nothing helps, you may want to talk to the doctor about medication to help an agitated person relax and sleep. Be aware that sleeping pills and tranquilizers may solve one problem and create another, such as sleeping at night but being more confused the next day.

Lewd Public Behavior

Sexually inappropriate behavior—undressing or masturbating in public or making unreasonable sexual demands or lewd remarks— may occur during the course of the illness. This behavior can be shocking and upsetting. It's important to remind yourself—and others—that it is caused by the disease.

Talk to your doctor about possible treatment plans. Meanwhile, develop an action plan to follow if the behavior occurs in certain situations. Decide what you will do if she undresses at home, outside of the home, or around other adults or children. Try to identify what triggers the behavior. Sometimes it is simply the fact that her clothing is making her uncomfortable.

Aggression

Aggressive behavior is one of the most unsettling and frightening symptoms of Alzheimer's disease. It can make caring for a loved one at home extremely difficult—and at times, potentially unsafe for everyone involved.

Fact

Outbursts tend to occur when a person is dressing, bathing, or at a doctor's appointment. In those situations, someone with Alzheimer's is more likely to misinterpret certain actions, grow anxious, and respond aggressively. Aggression can also be triggered by a physical illness such as constipation or infection, pain, depression or anxiety, or lack of sleep.

It's important that a doctor evaluate a patient to identify any physical complaints that may be contributing to the problem. Also keep in mind that establishing a routine may help people with dementia feel more at ease. "People with Alzheimer's do better when they have a routine," says AD specialist Eric Tangalos, MD. "It allows them to refresh and reinforce their pattern of behavior every day. They get to relearn their habits over and over and this is good."

Try to make difficult daily tasks easier—even pleasant—by doing them at a time when your loved one seems to be most calm and alert. Bathe in the morning, if that's her best time. Take a walk with her in the late afternoon if she gets aggravated then. Try making a routine more pleasant by playing some of her favorite music.

Regular and gentle exercise can help reduce agitation and aggressive behavior. If the behavior is ongoing and difficult, your doctor may prescribe medications to treat the problem.

Communicating Calmly

Improving your communication skills is one of the most effective ways to handle difficult behavior in people with dementia, according to the national Family Caregiver Alliance (FCA), a go-to source of information, advice, and referrals for the estimated 44 million Americans who provide unpaid care to another adult at home.

Better communication can make caregiving less stressful, improve the quality of your relationship, and enhance your ability to handle difficult behavior. Try these strategies:

1. Actions speak louder than words. If you are tense and upset—if your jaw is clenched or your sentences clipped—you convey those feelings and thoughts, not your words. Set a positive mood by speaking to your loved one in a pleasant and respectful manner. Show affection with facial expressions, tone of voice, and physical touch. It will make both of you feel better.
2. Limit distractions and noise—turn off the radio or TV, close the curtains, or shut the door. Move to quieter surroundings.
3. State your message clearly. Use simple words and sentences. Speak slowly, distinctly, and in a reassuring tone.

Pitch your voice lower, not higher. If she doesn't understand the first time, use the same wording to repeat what you said. Use the names of people and places instead of pronouns or abbreviations. (Ask "Did Dad go out?" not "Is he here?")

4. Ask simple questions that require simple yes or no responses. Refrain from asking open-ended questions or giving too many choices. ("Would you like to wear your white shirt or your blue shirt?" is far better than "What would you like to wear?") Visual cues (holding up an item of clothing) can help clarify your question and help her respond.

5. Listen with your ears, eyes, and heart. Be patient as you wait for your loved one's reply. If she is struggling for an answer, it's okay to suggest words. Watch for nonverbal cues and body language, and respond appropriately. Always try to listen for the meaning and feelings that underlie the words.

6. The best way to approach any large, complex activity is to break it down into a series of manageable tasks. For someone with AD, the many steps involved in getting ready for a doctor's appointment or making dinner can be overwhelming. Encourage her to do one thing at a time: get her clothes on, comb her hair, brush her teeth, feed the cat. Even these individual tasks are made up of many small steps that may be unmanageable. Gently remind her of steps she tends to forget. ("Have you got your purse?") Help with things she can't accomplish on her own. Using visual cues, such as showing her with your hand where to place the dinner plate, can be very helpful.

7. When the going gets tough, don't keep going. If your loved one becomes upset, try changing the subject or the environment. It is important to connect with the person emotionally, before you distract and redirect. "You seem sad," you might say. "I understand that. Let's go for a walk or get something to eat."

8. Respond with affection and reassurance. People with dementia often feel confused, anxious, and unsure of themselves. They confuse a movie or a memory with reality. Avoid pointing out that they're wrong. Clear up confusion only if and when it matters. ("Mom, I think you're hearing the phone ring on the TV show. Don't worry about the phone; the answering machine is on.") Stay focused on her feelings and responses, which are real. Reassure her, particularly if she saw something distressing on a TV show and is worried about it. Try holding hands, touching, hugging, or laughing about how "real" so much of what's on TV seems these days.

9. Talk about the good old days. Remembering the past can be soothing and affirming for people with dementia, who may better recall life at age forty-five than what happened forty-five minutes ago. Try to avoid asking questions that rely on her short-term memory, such as what she had for lunch or what your sister said when she called earlier.

10. Maintain your sense of humor. Use it as often as possible to laugh with (never at) her. Chances are, she'll be delighted to laugh along with you. People with dementia tend to retain their social skills and are usually happy to enjoy a good, healthy laugh.

Remember that, despite everything you do, you and your loved one are battling a relentless disease whose symptoms—including outbursts—will continue. When that happens, try your best to remain calm and defuse the situation. Knowing what you now know, you will get through it.

CHAPTER 15

Coping with Alzheimer's Day to Day

The medical, psychological, social, and institutional challenges of caring for someone with Alzheimer's are enormous. But helping a loved one cope with the basic activities of daily living, such as eating, dressing, and bathing, can be difficult and daunting as well. Trying to help a person with dementia maintain privacy and dignity requires thought, planning, and a sense of balance, especially as it becomes more difficult for her to care for herself.

Eating and Drinking

People with dementia frequently lose interest in food. They may miss meals, forget they've eaten, or eat whatever is on hand. Any or all of these behaviors can make mealtimes difficult. Poor nutrition can also compromise your loved one's health and well-being.

Establish a Mealtime Routine

Eating with someone who isn't hungry, pushes away foods, or becomes frustrated and upset is difficult and unpleasant for everyone at the table. Try to serve meals at the same time every day and limit distractions while you are eating. Turn off the TV, radio, and phone so you can focus on eating. Eat together. Make meals an enjoyable event so that your loved one looks forward to the experience.

Put out only the utensils you need for the meal. Try to serve only one or two foods at a time. Too many choices may be confusing.

Your loved one may develop a sudden craving for food she never cared about before and leave old favorites on her plate. Try to be flexible. If she doesn't eat enough—or if she's always hungry—make sure to have healthy finger foods such as fruit and vegetables on hand.

Avoid Food Hazards

Remember that people with dementia may have difficulty swallowing. Be careful if you serve popcorn, carrots, and nuts. All of these foods can get caught in the throat. You may want to avoid them altogether. Always be sure to check the temperature of food you serve, as your loved one might not realize something is too hot or cold.

Essential

Keep the table setting calm and simple. Put the candles, flowers, and condiments aside. Bottles of ketchup, sauce, salt, and pepper can confuse someone with AD. Set the table with simple, unpatterned plates that set off the color and texture of the food. People with dementia lose visual and spatial abilities, and they may have trouble distinguishing the food from the plate.

Manners and Mess

Once-fastidious people may start eating with their fingers, spilling things, and making a mess at the dinner table as their symptoms progress. If your loved one is sitting down and eating healthy meals, you may not care that she's making a mess. If it bothers you, consider these strategies:

- Use a plastic tablecloth or placemat for easier cleanup.
- Set the table with sturdy plastic dishes and cups.

- Use plastic smocks or aprons.
- Use knives, forks, and spoons with handles that are easy to manipulate. These are available in medical supply stores and catalogs, but you might also check for picnic and barbeque utensils.
- Use plates with suction cups to prevent sliding.
- Put plastic cloth on the floor for any spillage.

Essential

People with dementia gradually lose the ability to perform rote tasks like eating or combing their hair. In mid-stage dementia, you can offer cues, miming how to use a spoon or comb and reminding her what to do.

Thirst and Dehydration

Your body's ability to detect thirst diminishes with age. Older people and people with dementia are more likely than most to suffer serious dehydration. Typically, the problem is caused by not drinking enough liquid or excreting too much urine. But many illnesses and medications can also cause dehydration as well. Dehydration can cause headaches, dry mouth and tongue, and more serious conditions, including confusion and disorientation—the most common symptoms of dementia. Be sure your loved one drinks enough liquids every day.

Dressing

Dressing is difficult for most dementia patients. Choosing appropriate undergarments, clothes, and outerwear can cause anxiety, even panic, in someone who is confused. At the same time, she may shirk all advice, suggestions, and assistance in dressing herself.

Your first goal should be to devise a strategy that allows her to dress herself appropriately as long as she can, according to Coach Broyles. Start by surveying your mother's closet and drawers. Chances are, both are filled with clothes she no longer wears (evening clothes and business suits, for example), and accessories she won't wear as her illness progresses (high heels, panty hose, or even bras, which can be uncomfortable or hard to put on). Store or give away as much as possible.

Fact

Southeastern Conference football legend and Arkansas Razorbacks Coach Frank Broyles is the author of *Coach Broyles' Playbook for Alzheimer's Caregivers*. The playbook, available at no charge from the Alzheimer's Association, is based on Coach Broyles's experience caring for his late wife, who suffered from Alzheimer's disease.

Make sure all her clothes and shoes fit right. Sometimes, people with AD refuse to wear clothes or take them off in public because they're uncomfortable.

Group clothing into "outfits" that make it easier for her to dress herself, or for you or another caregiver to lay out. Allow a lot of time for her to get dressed. Compliment her good choices.

People with dementia tend to wear the same clothes over and over. If that's the case, buy duplicate outfits or clothes that look alike.

Grooming and Hygiene

A person with dementia may forget how to comb his hair, clip his fingernails, or brush his teeth. Try to maintain grooming routines. If he gets his hair cut by a barber, continue this as long as you can. If the experience becomes overwhelming, ask the barber to come to the home.

If your loved one seems overwhelmed, bewildered, or incapable of performing basic tasks, ask yourself these questions:

- ❑ Are there medical problems (such as depression) that could be making him listless and apathetic?
- ❑ Does he know what to do with a brush or a face cloth?
- ❑ Has he forgotten what he was doing before finishing a task?
- ❑ Is his vision impaired? What about his hearing?
- ❑ Does he have too many choices or decisions to make?
- ❑ Does your presence embarrass him?
- ❑ Are your instructions clear?

Oral Care

Don't neglect oral health in someone with dementia. Proper oral care is essential in preventing tooth decay and gum disease, both of which can discourage him from eating. Take him to the dentist.

⌷ Essential

Don't stress about your loved one getting dressed, experienced caregivers advise. The key is to rethink and simplify what she wears, when she wears it, and why. You can organize her wardrobe around clothes she likes to wear, particularly those that are comfortable and easy to put on and take off. (Think elastic waistbands; shoes with wide heels and Velcro fasteners.)

Remind him to brush twice a day with a soft-bristled toothbrush and fluoridated toothpaste. If he wears dentures, make sure they fit well, and clean them properly.

Grooming Tips

Women may need help applying makeup, but may enjoy doing so. Try to simplify and allow her to do as much as possible for herself. For some women, manicures, pedicures, and other skin treatments may provide some pleasure.

Ⳑ. Essential

Break down every personal task into simple steps and encourage him to do as many of them as possible. Do not rush the task; allow plenty of time. Try to give visual cues as well as verbal instructions. Hand him a toothbrush, for example, when you tell him it's time to brush his teeth. Demonstrate, if it helps.

Men should use an electric razor, and try to shave at a regular time of day, or when he seems most willing. If shaving becomes too difficult, let the beard grow.

Bathing

Bathing is frequently a fraught issue for people with AD and family caretakers. With reason: As children, most of us are taught that using the toilet and bathing ourselves are private, personal activities. Being undressed and cleaned by another adult can be embarrassing, distressing, and even humiliating for both caregivers and their loved ones.

The difficulty is sometimes exacerbated by mistaken beliefs, according to dementia care experts at the University of North Carolina, whose book and website, *Bathing Without a Battle*, dispels "myths about bathing." Go to *www.bathingwithoutabattle.unc.edu* for more information. If your loved one needs you to take charge of his hygiene routine, consider what is likely to make him feel most familiar—and comfortable—with the process.

Be Mindful—and Flexible

Rethink your assumptions about bathing and cleanliness and adjust them to the situation. Is it necessary to shower or bathe every day, or is twice a week sufficient? How often must his hair be washed? Is dry shampoo an option?

L. Essential

Ask yourself: What would make him feel more comfortable and relaxed about this process? Has he always taken baths or showers? Bathed in the morning or at night? Incorporating as many aspects of his own routine into a new one should provide some comfort and help him preserve his dignity.

Older people in particular are afraid of slipping and falling. Is the bathroom well lit, comfortable, and equipped with nonslip floor bath mats, grab bars, and bath or shower seats? What about a hand-held shower? Have all the bath things you need laid out beforehand. If you are giving your loved one a bath, draw the water first. Check the temperature of the water.

If your loved one has always been modest, respect that and make sure doors and curtains are closed. Drape him in a large towel, lifting it to wash as needed. Have towels and a robe or his clothes ready when he gets out.

If bathing in the tub or shower is too traumatic for your loved one, try a towel bath. Dampen a large bath towel and washcloths in a plastic bag filled with warm water and no-rinse soap. Use an extra-large towel or bath blanket to keep your loved one covered, dry, and warm while you clean and massage him with the dampened towel and washcloths.

Incontinence

People lose control of their bladders and bowels more frequently as dementia progresses. But some accidents happen because they forget where the bathroom is located or can't get to it in time. And some of those instances can be prevented.

If your loved one wets or soils herself, try to minimize her embarrassment and help maintain her dignity. Then establish a routine for using the toilet.

Try reminding her to use the bathroom every two hours and assist her if necessary. Encourage her to wear easy-to-remove, washable clothing with elastic waistbands. While making sure she doesn't become dehydrated, you should also avoid drinks with a diuretic effect, including coffee, tea, soda, and beer.

Alert

Never leave a person with dementia unattended in the bath or shower. The chances of her slipping and falling, frightening or hurting herself, or hitting her head are too great to take any risks.

Limit how much liquid she drinks before bedtime, and remember that people become more confused than usual when they wake during the night. Put up signs (with illustrations) showing which door leads to the bathroom. If it's far from where she sleeps, you may want to purchase a commode to leave in the bedroom at night for easy access.

You also may want to buy incontinence pads and products that are now available at any pharmacy or supermarket.

Wandering

More than 60 percent of people with dementia wander at some point, according to the Alzheimer's Association. In other words, nearly anyone with AD is at risk. Someone may be at higher risk if he comes home later than usual from his customary walk or drive, tries to go home when he is already home, or wants to get to work even though he's retired. Wandering is also common among people who appear restless, or who continually look for familiar objects and people they think they have lost.

The side effects of medication can lead to wandering. So can stress, anxiety, and confusion. People with AD grow increasingly confused about the time of day, day of the week, and season of the year. They have trouble recognizing family, friends, and familiar household objects (a fork, a toothbrush, a phone). They misinterpret what they see or hear.

Question

What is it about AD that makes people walk aimlessly, sometimes for hours?
Caregiving pros at FCA say, "They may be bored, bothered, or searching for 'something' or someone. They may be trying to fulfill a physical need—thirst, hunger, a need to use the toilet, or exercise. Discovering the triggers for wandering are not always easy, but they can provide insights to dealing with the behavior."

Because any number of AD symptoms and treatments can encourage episodes of wandering, you should take steps to discourage it even if it hasn't yet happened.

❏ Be sure he gets regular exercise and activity; this can discourage restlessness.
❏ Install locks that require you to use a key. Position locks high or low on the door; many people with dementia don't look beyond eye level. (However, don't forget fire and safety concerns for all family members.)
❏ Put child-safe plastic covers on your doorknobs.
❏ Think about putting in a home security or home monitoring system.
❏ Don't let him sit around doing nothing or watching TV. Movement—and exercise in particular—reduces anxiety and agitation.

❑ Make sure his basic needs are met. Check to see if he might be hungry, thirsty, or need to use the bathroom.

❑ Keep him involved in any household activities he can handle.

❑ Reassure him if he feels lost, abandoned, or disoriented. ("This store is really crowded. I can't wait to get home.")

❑ Makes sure his coat, hat, and keys are put away.

❑ Keep a recent picture of him on hand to show neighbors or the police if necessary.

Sources: *Alzheimer's Association; ADEAR*

Fact

Consider enrolling in the Alzheimer's Association MedicAlert + Safe Return membership program. One phone call alerts public safety officials, the local Alzheimer's Association, and medical emergency responders that someone is lost. You can enroll in the program for $49.95 with a $25 annual renewal fee by calling 888-572-8566 or visiting the Alzheimer's Association website (*www.alz.org*).

Distress over wandering episodes frequently convinces caregivers to move loved ones to a nursing home or another supervised setting, according to AD experts.

Travel

Think ahead if you plan to travel with someone who has Alzheimer's disease. Think about her needs over the course of two days, and how you can meet them on a car trip or in an airport, someone else's home, or a hotel.

If she hasn't traveled recently and you're planning a trip that will last more than a few days, you may want to try taking a short trip to see how she responds.

Essential

Be sure to consider the stage of your loved one's illness. Change makes many people with AD anxious and can cause agitation and aggression. Think about her behavioral symptoms, which may be affected by traveling away from home.

Here are a few other suggestions to keep in mind:

- ❑ Consider planning trips and vacations at a place that is familiar to her; a lake cabin or inn she has visited in the past, for example.
- ❑ If your loved one isn't familiar with plane travel, consider driving or taking a train. If you do fly, alert the airlines you are traveling with a person who is memory impaired.
- ❑ Make certain she is carrying or wearing some sort of identification in case she gets lost.
- ❑ Avoid crowds if your loved one is easily agitated.
- ❑ Plan to move slowly. This is probably not the right time for a jam-packed visit to extended family or a fast-paced sight-seeing trip.
- ❑ Never leave a person with dementia alone in a car. When you're moving, be sure to keep her seat belt buckled and the doors locked.
- ❑ Plan regular rest stops.
- ❑ If your loved one becomes agitated while traveling in a car, stop at the first available place. Never try to calm down a person while you are driving.
- ❑ Plan simple travel activities for someone with Alzheimer's disease. Reading a magazine, playing with a deck of cards, or listening to music can help keep your loved one calm when traveling.

AD patients don't do well in strange surroundings, which is why travel, visiting out-of-town family for the holidays, or going to a hospital can be very difficult for someone with the disease, according to Eric Tangalos, MD. He adds, "A change in routine is not good for people with Alzheimer's—there are just too many problems to try and solve."

Fact

You take your caregiving responsibilities with you when you're on vacation. Chances are, the job may be more demanding in an unfamiliar setting. Consider taking someone with you who can and will help you with these duties.

Day-to-Day Basics

A key to successful caregiving is problem solving. The more you understand AD, the easier it is to find solutions to daily care dilemmas.

In Alzheimer's, the part of the brain that controls sequencing is damaged. That's why your loved one may have trouble putting on clothing in the right order. If the part of his brain that initiates an activity is damaged, he will probably need help starting a task like eating or brushing his teeth. People with dementia sometimes look at an item, such as a hairbrush, and are not able to recognize it.

QUICK TIPS ON DAILY CARE FROM THE ALZHEIMER'S ASSOCIATION

1. Be flexible. Adapt to the person's preferences.
2. Help the person stay as independent as possible.
3. Guide by using easy, step-by-step directions.
4. Speak in short and simple words.
5. Avoid rushing the person through a task.

6. Encourage, reassure, and praise the person.
7. Watch for unspoken communication.
8. Experiment with new approaches.
9. Consider using different types of products such as bathing chairs or large-grip toothbrushes.
10. Be patient, understanding, and sensitive.

Some days, grooming routines go smoothly. On others, they're a tremendous challenge. On those days, decide what's worth the effort and what isn't. Adequate clothing and basic hygiene may be enough on some days. Remember: you are doing the best you can.

A FAMILY DISEASE

"You really can't imagine how consuming caring for someone with dementia can be," says Amy, whose father is caring for her mother, who has AD.

"My mother's care is a twenty-four-hour-a-day, seven-day-a-week job that's consuming my father, an eighty-six-year-old retiree with health problems of his own. People with Alzheimer's need care and attention just to stay safe all day long and at night. My mother is up and down at all hours, and neither of them sleep.

"He's better off than many people. He's got family close by, and we give him some support on evenings and weekends.

"But he really needs in-home health care, and he's resistant to it. I think he's afraid to trust someone else in their home with her care.

"He can't get out to buy milk or a newspaper. She has to go with him. And he can't leave her alone when they go out together.

"There was an episode recently, when she went into the ladies room by herself and didn't come back. There was no one around, so he went in to check on her and found her crying, helpless. She'd missed the toilet and there was a major mess on the floor.

"This was devastating for both of them, and it showed some of the simple things people need, like family bathrooms at malls and other public places.

"No one really knows what to do in that situation, which is why Alzheimer's is difficult for the whole family. Education and coping mechanisms for the caregiver are as critical as any medications the patient receives."

CHAPTER 16

Treatments on the Horizon

Our understanding of Alzheimer's has grown exponentially during the past two decades. But sophisticated knowledge has yet to yield effective diagnostic tools or treatments, much less a cure for the disease. Alzheimer's, like cancer, is a "complex pathologic process" that involves genetic, biological, and environmental factors, according to Ronald Petersen, MD, director of the Mayo Clinic Alzheimer's Disease Research Center. Scientists are now studying and targeting elements of that complex pathology with the hope of developing a combination of strategies to combat the disease.

Curing Alzheimer's: A Cautionary Tale

Traveling on assignment in March 2007, NBC News chief science and health correspondent Robert Bazell received a fusillade of frantic voice and e-mail messages from editors trumpeting "a cure for Alzheimer's disease!" The source of the excitement was Myriad Genetics, a biotechnology company then testing an experimental drug called Flurizan, which had shown some promise of treating memory loss and other AD symptoms in Phase II clinical trials that had ended in 2006. The drug was being tested in Phase III trials, slated to end in 2008. Meanwhile, a company press release boasted more good news about Flurizan, describing it as a drug that "may be capable, not only of slowing the decline of Alzheimer's disease, but of halting the disease in its tracks." Myriad Genetics cited no data for these incredible claims, which several small media outlets reported as breakthrough news nonetheless.

Bazell, a veteran medical reporter who questions and verifies information before reporting it as fact, checked with the Alzheimer's Association and trustworthy Alzheimer's researchers to see if this was "dramatic, unexpected new research" or "yet another case of biotechnology hype." It was the latter, as it so often is, Bazell wrote later in his "Second Opinion" column on MSNBC.com. Bazell notes that only rarely does something entirely unexpected happen in science. Scientific and clinical studies proceed slowly and methodically, and their progress is reported in medical journals and by organizations like the Alzheimer's Association.

Myriad put out a press release to tell the world that 42 percent of forty-three patients who had done well in the Phase II Flurizan trial did not get any worse during the subsequent year. A study of forty-three people is too small to reveal anything—much less a breakthrough in treatment for an intractable disease, Bazell pointed out.

Research and development of Flurizan stopped in its tracks the following year, when Phase III clinical trials showed the drug did not improve thinking and memory skills or the ability to carry out everyday tasks in a study of 1,700 men and women with mild cognitive impairment.

Disappointing Drug Experiments

Flurizan is one of a handful of Alzheimer's treatments whose red-hot hopes went cold once they reached the final phases of clinical (human) study.

Shortly before Myriad Genetics gave up on Flurizan, British researchers announced that an experimental vaccine designed to eliminate the amyloid plaques thought to cause dementia had worked—but not the way it was supposed to. Researchers followed sixty-four patients with moderate Alzheimer's for an average of six years in the vaccine study, during which nine patients died of Alzheimer's disease. Autopsies of those patients showed that nearly all plaque was gone from their brains. Nevertheless, those patients had still developed severe dementia; the toxic plaques were gone, but the disease was not.

Essential

Most scientists ascribe to what's known as the amyloid hypothesis, which maintains that Alzheimer's centers on the overproduction of beta-amyloid plaques that build up between nerve cells in the brain. Some scientists believe that twisted fibers of the protein tau (neurofibrillary tangles) that accumulate inside cells and cause their collapse are the fundamental culprit in AD.

The trial was one of a growing number of studies that have caused some scientists to question whether the cause-effect relationship between amyloid and dementia is as straightforward as Alzheimer science has long assumed. Researchers, who still aren't sure if plaque is a cause or an effect of AD, are learning that an overabundance of plaques, an Alzheimer's hallmark, are less telling a symptom than is widely believed.

Drug Therapies

Researchers are pressing ahead with pharmaceuticals aimed at an array of targets. Some attack different phases of plaque formation; others immunize the body against amyloid.

The more promising in late-stage investigative trials include the following:

- **Rember.** Rember is the first drug that directly attacks the tau protein tangles that form inside nerve cells in the brain and impair concentration and memory, scientists say. The tangles first destroy the nerve cells linked to memory and then proceed to attack neurons in other parts of the brain. Researchers believe Rember may arrest that progression.
- **Bapineuzumab.** Large clinical trials in the United States and Canada are studying this immunotherapy treatment for mild to moderate AD. Bapineuzumab is designed to provide antibodies against amyloid-beta peptides directly to the patient. Those antibodies can bind to and remove amyloid peptide from the brain, eliminating plaque and inhibiting the damage it does, scientists say.
- **Dimebon.** Originally developed and marketed in Russia as an antihistamine, Dimebon has emerged as a potential treatment for Alzheimer's, Huntington's disease, and other neurodegenerative diseases. Dimebon stabilized Alzheimer's disease for at least eighteen months in a Russian study. Patient participants treated with the drug were reported to have better or not-much-worse mental function than patients who were given placebo pills, whose symptoms got significantly worse.

Fact

Recent brain imaging research and population studies show that some people accumulate significant plaques and tangles without developing cognitive impairment. Explanations of this vary, but some maintain that people with extra "brain reserve" may be more resistant to dementia symptoms, including characteristic Alzheimer's pathology.

However, Alzheimer's experts such as Gary J. Kennedy, MD, director of geriatric psychiatry at New York's Montefiore Medical Center, warn that placebo-treated Alzheimer's patients in Russia get different care than do U.S. patients. That difference could make any effect of Dimebon seem greater compared with placebo. Kennedy notes, too, that patients' actual improvement on Dimebon is not very different from improvement seen with the existing Alzheimer's drugs Aricept, Razadyne, and Exelon. Although well-respected Alzheimer's researchers from the United States were involved in the study, its results must be replicated by independent investigators in American and Western European settings before it receives approval.

Statins
Some studies of statins, cholesterol-lowering drugs, indicate that using these medications regularly in midlife decreases AD risk. But a large, eighteen-month study of the statin Lipitor showed it provided no cognitive or functional benefit to AD patients taking the drug.

 Alert

In the world of Alzheimer's treatment, where drugs currently approved to treat the illness offer some patients modest symptom relief for a year or less, the possibility of stabilizing patients for more than twelve months is viewed as a major breakthrough.

Nonsteroidal Anti-Inflammatory Drugs
Inflammation seems to occur frequently in the brains of some people with Alzheimer's, and several studies have looked at the effects of anti-inflammatory drugs such as ibuprofen (e.g., Advil), naproxen (e.g., Aleve), and indomethacin (e.g., Indocin) in treating or preventing AD. No anti-inflammatory has proven effective, though research continues.

Estrogen

Estrogen acts as a brain lubricant, and there is some evidence that estrogen supplements can nourish brain health in post-menopausal women, whose natural estrogen levels decline. Starting in the 1970s, synthetic estrogen therapy—sometimes called hormone replacement therapy—became available to women of menopausal age and older. The hormone was considered a palliative plus: a generally safe, effective treatment for menopause symptoms that seemed to help protect bones, veins, brains, and perhaps even the hearts of women over fifty. All that changed in 2002 when the federally commissioned and funded Women's Health Initiative announced it was halting a major clinical trial of a form of synthetic hormone replacement therapy after finding that its use slightly elevated the risk for breast cancer, heart disease, stroke, and blood clots among older women in the study. What's more, rather than protecting cognitive health, the study found that in women over sixty-five, an estrogen-progestin drug doubled the risk of dementia, possibly because the clotting effects of the drug impeded blood flow in the brain.

Fact

Despite promising leads, new treatments for Alzheimer's have been slow to emerge. Some AD specialists predict that many future treatments will focus on stopping the disease in people at risk. Some researchers predict that Alzheimer's will eventually be treated with a drug cocktail or a multiple-step process, much the same way combination chemotherapy is administered.

Subsequent research results suggest that estrogen actually does offer health benefits—and may improve cognitive function—in younger women (ages forty-five to fifty-five) if taken for a short time. In other words, the jury is out on whether estrogen protects against dementia.

Finding New Pathways

Alzheimer's investigations are hampered by a lack of sophisticated diagnostic tests that can detect the disease in its early stages. Absent such tools, Lewy body dementia and vascular dementia may be misdiagnosed as Alzheimer's disease.

Alzheimer's is currently diagnosed based on symptoms, cognitive testing, and a process of elimination—imprecise and relatively unsophisticated methods that may miss early signs of dementia, delaying detection and treatment until after irreversible damage has occurred. Researchers are searching for ways of identifying people at risk for dementia while they are still cognitively normal, so they can steer them toward trials and treatments and develop new therapies to help people preserve normal function. Brain changes that occur with Alzheimer's, including amyloid plaques and neurofibrillary tangles, begin developing years before abnormal clinical symptoms such as memory loss develop.

Fact

Because Alzheimer's pathology begins to develop long before symptoms appear, drugs that might prevent the disease would have to be taken for many years. These drugs have to be safe, carefully targeted, and cause minimal side effects, according to experts at the Alzheimer's Disease Genetics Initiative.

Development of increasingly sensitive, sophisticated imaging techniques has yielded encouraging results, and Alzheimer's scientists have trained energy and attention on using these technologies with biomarkers—a feature or facet present in the body that can be used to measure the progress of disease or the effects of treatment. Researchers hope these advances will lead to diagnostic tests that can help detect the disease before its symptoms appear and evaluate early interventions.

Imaging Technology

Scientists have already developed magnetic resonance imaging (MRI) and positron emission tomography (PET) scans that can identify and measure shrinkage and other signs of AD symptoms in the brain. Using positron emission tomography (PET) scanners, scientists can now "image" beta-amyloid plaque deposits in the brains of patients who have been injected with a radioactive compound or tracer. The tracer attaches to amyloid, which "lights up" when it is imaged in a PET scan of the brain. Other researchers are using computer analyses of MRI scans to assess the severity of AD-related neurofibrillary tangles.

Biomarkers in Clinical Trials

Researchers say that identifying biomarkers from blood or urine samples, which are easy to obtain, should lead to the development of simple blood tests that could be useful in detecting AD, assessing brain damage, and evaluating the effectiveness of therapies during clinical trials. Several noninvasive tests are in development, and some research scientists are hopeful that presymptomatic biomarkers can be used as "surrogates" for Alzheimer's disease to measure the effect of drugs on disease progression in clinical trials.

Because Alzheimer's progresses so slowly, it is often difficult to gauge the effectiveness of experimental drugs in Phase II clinical trials, which typically last no longer than eighteen months. Alzheimer's symptoms can't be readily diagnosed, and researchers have difficulty determining whether the drug has some real effect in studies that last less than two years. If a biomarker study could somehow measure clinical efficacy, research teams would know better which treatments should proceed to Phase III clinical trials.

However, some knowledgeable observers of Alzheimer's science question how useful biomarkers will be in clinical research in the next few years. After all, no biomarker can yet predict or diagnose Alzheimer's with scientific accuracy. Furthermore, neuroimaging studies suggesting that the presence or absence of amyloid plaques in the brain does not necessarily correspond with cognitive impairment call into question how valuable the diagnostics that detect amyloid plaques actually are.

Mild Cognitive Impairment

Some researchers are focusing on moving the "detection threshold" for AD to earlier stages by studying the earliest form of detectable dementia: mild cognitive impairment (MCI). Not everyone with MCI develops Alzheimer's, but the condition is regarded as a significant risk factor. The ranks of people diagnosed with mild cognitive impairment, already large, are growing.

Combination Therapies

Studies show that certain medications prescribed to treat other conditions may affect symptoms of AD. In one study, Alzheimer's patients who had diabetes and took insulin plus another anti-diabetes medication to control blood sugar had 80 percent fewer amyloid plaques. Researchers speculated that the drugs may normalize the brain's communication network of insulin receptors, which goes awry in people with Alzheimer's, while clearing away the damaging plaques in the brain.

Gene Therapy

Scientists are proceeding apace on gene research that may lead to clues about the causes and effective treatments of AD.

In the years to come, as researchers learn more about the human genome, they expect to find up to a dozen genetic abnormalities that predispose some people to late-onset Alzheimer's.

Significance of the ApoE4 Gene

As explained in Chapter 5, the ApoE gene codes for a protein that helps carry cholesterol in the bloodstream.

Scientists think learning more about the role of ApoE4 and other risk factor genes in the development of AD may help them identify who would benefit from prevention and treatment efforts, according to the National Institutes on Aging (NIA). The agency has launched a major study to discover any remaining genetic risk factors for late-onset AD. Geneticists from the institute's Alzheimer's Disease Centers are working to collect genetic samples from families affected by multiple cases of late-onset AD.

A blood test can identify which ApoE alleles you carry. But because the ApoE4 gene is only a risk factor for AD, the test can't tell you with any certainty if you will develop AD. Not everyone with ApoE4 develops Alzheimer's. Nor does everyone with Alzheimer's carry a copy of the ApoE4 variation. In some cases, ApoE testing is used in combination with other medical tests to strengthen the diagnosis of a suspected case of AD.

 Alert

The NIA warns that ApoE testing raises ethical, legal, and social questions. Confidentiality laws protect information gathered for research purposes. However, the information may not remain confidential if it becomes part of a person's medical records. Thereafter, employers, insurance companies, and other health care organizations could obtain genetic test results and use them to discriminate against job-seekers, employees and people seeking insurance coverage.

ApoE testing is part of the protocol in some clinical trials, and research volunteers may be able to learn the results of the test. Because the significance of the results depends on several other factors, the results can be complex and emotionally upsetting. The NIA and the Alzheimer's Association urge research study volunteers who opt to take the test and learn its results to get genetic counseling before and after testing.

Recent Gene Research

Early in 2007, fourteen teams of international researchers announced that variations of a gene called SORL1, which appear to increase the production of amyloid-beta plaques inside the brain, are associated with an increased rate of late-onset AD. The following year, researchers at Harvard Medical School and Massachusetts General Hospital identified four new genes that may increase the risk of the late-onset AD. One of the four appears to influence the age of Alzheimer's onset. A second gene causes a movement disorder called spinocerebellar ataxia; a third is involved in the innate immune system (part of the body's defense against bacteria and viruses); and a fourth gene produces a brain protein.

Scientists believe that understanding more about the genetic bases of Alzheimer's will help them better understand the mechanisms of the disease—how it begins and why some people with memory problems develop AD while others do not. They are eager to learn how AD risk factor genes interact with environmental and lifestyle factors to influence individual AD risk.

Genetic tests and screenings may eventually help identify people at high risk for AD and help them get early treatment, according to the National Institute on Aging (NIA). Genetic research may also lead to new approaches to prevention and treatment.

CHAPTER 17

Treating Alzheimer's Symptoms Without Drugs or Supplements

Lifestyle changes that may delay the development of dementia—exercising your brain and body, staying connected to family and friends, and eating a heart-healthy diet—may also help soothe some symptoms of Alzheimer's disease. None of these measures is a proven deterrent. But nondrug treatments from behavior modification to bright light are generally free of side effects, and they have been shown to improve health and quality of life for patients and caregivers alike.

Lightening the Burden of Alzheimer's

Dementia patients suffer from an incurable disease. Many are further burdened by "excess disability"—depression, agitation, sleep disturbances, or physical problems such as falling—that impairs their overall health and well-being and may even speed their cognitive decline.

For years, it was widely believed nothing could help people with AD. More recently, clinicians have developed and tested a variety of nondrug interventions that can increase patients' physical activity, decrease their disability, improve mood, and, perhaps, delay the need for institutionalization.

"Just because you have a broken leg doesn't mean you have to drag around a ball and chain," says Dr. Linda Teri, a pioneer in nonpharmaceutical care and treatment for Alzheimer's at the University of Washington, Seattle. She likens dementia to a broken leg and the ball and chain to excess disability. Even if you can't cure dementia, you can take away the ball and chain and make it easier for the patient to walk around. Teri encourages caregivers to use flexible, individualized approaches to behavior modification strategies in home and institutional settings.

BRIGHT CAREGIVING MOMENTS

Like many dedicated caregivers, Bob DeMarco has a hard time keeping his mother socialized. If it were up to her, "she would sit around all day in the dark, rarely speaking," DeMarco writes in his popular blog, the Alzheimer's Reading Room (*www.alzheimersreadingroom.com*).

One Friday night, he decided to take his mother out to the Banana Boat in Boynton Beach, Florida—an outdoor restaurant and bar on the Intercoastal Waterway. Bob's mother rarely speaks when they go out to dinner, so he decided they would sit at the bar, eat, and listen to the live band. They went the next Friday and the Friday after. She seemed to like the routine.

"After a few weeks, women started to come over and talk to us. The attraction was an older man with his elderly mother; they wanted to say how nice it was to see us," he recalls.

"After a while, a small group of people started saving a chair for my mother as they were expecting us. As time went on, our little group of friends started to get bigger." They became real friends and started sharing birthdays and other happy occasions. DeMarco calls it a godsend.

But something close to a miracle occurred one Friday night. Bob's mom loves to dance. "Each and every week I asked her if she wanted to dance. Our new friends would also ask Mom to dance—men and women alike. I could tell that

Mom wanted to dance, but she always said no. Mom is no longer confident around crowds or people she doesn't know."

One Friday, as they got up to leave, Bob started dancing with her right on the spot. "She was shaking it a little bit and had a big smile on her face," he writes. "By the time we were done people had tears in their eyes and smiles as big as big could be.

"I have a vivid image of the look on Mom's face and of us dancing. I will have that image in my mind forever."

Engaging in pleasant activities can help alleviate depression in people with AD. However, what's enjoyable to an avid baseball fan may not appeal to his friend the classical music lover. Like most people, AD patients are more likely to engage in things they have always enjoyed. Teri and her colleagues have developed a pleasant activities checklist of activities such as baseball, classical music, gardening and card playing to start caregivers thinking about what might be helpful in encouraging patients to engage.

Essential

People with Alzheimer's gradually lose the ability to communicate. Try to identify what triggers difficult behavior, which is frequently set off by changes in environment, such as a new caregiver, houseguests, a change in living arrangements, or being asked to bathe, shower, or change clothes. Identify the symptom, understand its cause, and change the environment.

Similarly, the environmental triggers that set off difficult behavior in people with dementia vary from person to person. Teri and her colleagues urge caregivers to try an "ABC" approach to reducing behavioral problems: identify A (the activator or antecedent) that sets off B (behavior) and results in C (consequences). If you can understand the particular sequence of events that leads to someone's agitation, you may be able to defuse or even eliminate causes of the problem.

Exercise: The Proven Brain and Body Booster

Exercise enhances cognitive function more than any diet, drug, supplement, or brain stimulation therapy does currently. Aerobic exercise increases blood volume and promotes new cell growth in aging brains, and that cell growth improves memory. Exercise also increases the amount of the chemical BDNF (brain-derived neurotrophic factor) circulating in the brain, stimulating the birth and growth of new brain cells. Recent research indicates that vigorous physical activity actually protects against brain shrinkage in people with early-stage AD.

Essential

If your loved one insists he isn't healthy enough to exercise, consider asking your doctor to write him a prescription for a regular walk or exercise class. Studies have shown that exercise helps slow the deterioration of areas of the brain that are responsible for memory.

At a time when someone is losing skills in every aspect of her adult life, developing and improving physical ability can be very rewarding. Swimming an extra lap, walking a little further, or feeling strong enough to get around without a walker are tangible gains that can be a source of pride—both for the person with Alzheimer's and her caregivers.

Before you begin any exercise program, check with your doctor about:

- The best types of exercise and those to avoid
- How hard to work out

- How long to work out
- Possible referrals to other professionals, such as a physical therapist, who can help create a personal exercise program.

Multiple Benefits

Physical exercise—gentle stretching, strength training, balance, and endurance—is critical to maintaining strength and mobility in all older adults. People with Alzheimer's have a higher risk of falls and fractures than do people the same age without the disease. Once injured, they're also more likely to re-injure themselves—a pattern that can impede independence. Even a moderate amount of exercise improves strength and coordination, and that can reduce the risk of falls and injury.

Fact

Recent research shows that organized exercise designed to increase strength, flexibility, mobility, and coordination can improve overall physical function among nursing home patients with AD. A Spanish study showed that patients who exercised developed strength, agility, and endurance and were better able to perform daily activities.

Sleep disturbances are common among people with Alzheimer's disease, and physical activity is a natural sleep enhancer. Taking a daily walk or exercise class can help a person with AD relax more before bedtime, reduce agitation, and discourage nighttime wandering and fitful sleeping.

Exercise is also a proven antidote to high blood pressure, high cholesterol, and diabetes—all common health problems among older people.

Getting Going with Exercise

Starting an exercise program is hard for most people. It is particularly difficult for someone in the early stages of AD, who has a hard time starting and staying with a new routine or behavior. As AD progresses, people also tend to have trouble learning and recalling directions.

Because exercise benefits both patients and caregivers alike, why not exercise together? Check with your local Alzheimer's Association office, health center, or senior center for exercise programs geared to people living with Alzheimer's and other dementias.

Walking with another person outdoors is a safe, beneficial way for someone with AD to get exercise. In inclement weather, you can head for a local mall. Many indoor, climate-controlled shopping centers have programs for mall walkers. Even if yours doesn't, chances are you'll find other people interested in strolling and chatting when you go.

Move to Boost Your Mood

As many as 70 percent of people diagnosed with AD also have symptoms of depression, a condition that, if untreated, can exacerbate cognitive decline. People who are depressed lose interest in doing things they once enjoyed. Exercise helps discourage this tendency. In one survey of people with Alzheimer's, those who engaged in just sixty minutes of moderate exercise per week had reduced rates of depression after three months. Among members of a control group of who did not exercise, symptoms got worse over the same period.

Holding Steady

Over the course of a four-year Rush University study, elders who consistently engaged in mentally stimulating activities were 47 percent less likely to be diagnosed with Alzheimer's disease than were those who reported participating in a few mentally challenging activities.

Mental stimulation doesn't depend on years of education or degrees earned. Anything that exercises your brain—reading, doing crossword puzzles, woodworking, or trying a new hobby—nourishes nerve cells and the connections among them, say dementia specialists. The key to building brainpower is to challenge your brain with new tasks and processes.

Fact

Happy people spend a lot of time socializing, going to church, and reading newspapers; unhappy people spend a lot of time watching television. Sociologists reached these conclusions based on the responses of 45,000 Americans, which were collected over thirty-five years by the University of Chicago's General Social Survey.

Try square dancing, chess, tai chi, yoga, or sculpture. Working with modeling clay helps develop agility and eye-hand coordination. Playing bingo regularly bolsters the eye-hand connection—and adds the benefit of socializing. Dancing combines physical activity and mental activity; dancers are required to remember dance steps and coordinate them with a partner's steps. It has been associated with significantly reduced cognitive decline among older adults.

Cognitive Rehabilitation

Interest in cognitive training, or brain exercise, and cognitive rehabilitation has boomed in recent years, as baby boomers and healthy seniors seek ways of sharpening their memories and minds.

Early studies of brain-training in people with early Alzheimer's show that cognitive stimulation programs, which typically involve memory exercises and games designed to ramp up overall brain activity, may be less helpful than cognitive rehabilitation, according to Dr. David A. Loewenstein, professor of psychiatry and behavioral sciences at the University of Miami School of Medicine.

Cognitive rehabilitation, which is typically used to treat brain injuries and to help older adults recover from traumas like heart attacks and strokes, can help people with mild Alzheimer's improve their ability to perform specific tasks. Cognitive rehab isn't ready-made for treating Alzheimer's, acknowledges Loewenstein, who explains that AD progressively damages parts of the brain employed in many standard rehabilitation techniques.

Fact

Conversation may sharpen memory as much as brain games! Socializing—even talking to someone for ten minutes—was found to boost memory and stimulate the mind just as much as mental exercise, electronic games, and puzzles among seniors who took part in a 2007 University of Michigan study.

But while people with early stage Alzheimer's may have problems with explicit memory—knowledge of facts, knowing what happened when—they tend to retain their implicit or procedural memory—skills involved in eating and grooming, for example. Developing preserved procedural memory may help in cognitive rehabilitation.

Complementary Therapies

Nontraditional treatments that are used in addition to conventional therapies are sometimes called complementary care. With any alternative treatment you consider, find out if the potential benefits outweigh the risks.

Acupuncture

Elemental to traditional Chinese medicine, acupuncture has shown promise in treating mood problems and anxiety in small, scientific studies at the Wellesley College Center for Research on Women and at the University of Hong Kong. The Hong Kong study showed cognitive improvement among eight people with AD treated for thirty days with acupuncture. While this was a very small sample size, researchers are further investigating the effectiveness of acupuncture for treating mood and behavioral disturbances associated with Alzheimer's disease.

Aromatherapy

Flower and plant oils have been used for centuries to soothe the mind and body. One British study showed that lemon balm reduced agitation in people with Alzheimer's. Some patients and caregivers have experimented with lavender oil, which is thought to aid relaxation, and jasmine, which may boost alertness. Some eldercare facilities use aromatherapy to help calm residents. However, it is worth noting that many people with Alzheimer's lose their sense of smell as the disease progresses.

Art Therapy

Walking through a museum or gallery and looking at photos, paintings, or sculpture can be pleasant and stimulating, particularly for someone who is having difficulty with language and communication. Many people with dementia also enjoy working on art projects.

Bright Light Therapy

Recent studies of bright light therapy suggest it may be useful in lifting mood and aiding sleep in people with AD. Environmental light affects your body's twenty-four-hour biological clock (also known as the circadian rhythm), and too little light exposure can throw off that sensitive balance. Since the 1980s, mental health professionals have recommended bright light therapy to people suffering a depression known as seasonal affective disorder (SAD), which is thought to occur in people whose bodies produce excess melatonin—a hormone that helps control body temperature and sleep—during low-light months in the fall and winter. Some studies show that exposure to bright light can suppress the brain's production of melatonin, help regulate your body's internal clock, and lift mood.

Fact

Recent research shows that "elderspeak"—the overly familiar, infantilizing way in which caregivers, friends, and family sometimes address seniors—irritates and upsets people with AD. That discourages patients from cooperating and diminishes the quality of care in clinical and institutional settings such as nursing homes. Experts advise caregivers to speak in simple, straightforward sentences rather than using baby talk.

As we age, our eyes let in less light, and researchers theorize this can lead older patients' bodies to produce more melatonin. Increasing patients' exposure to natural light can be as simple as going for a walk outside first thing in the morning. Light therapy for Alzheimer's patients may help improve mood and realign the body's internal clock.

Massage

Massage can help relieve muscle tension, promote relaxation, and alleviate anxiety and stress. Massage can also cause your body to release natural painkillers, and it may boost your immune system, according to medical authorities. Though few studies have been done on massage for Alzheimer's patients, some caregivers believe it can reduce episodes of wandering and other agitated behaviors. Massage can also help people with the disease sleep better.

Music Therapy

Older adults with Alzheimer's disease and other memory disorders have been treated successfully with music therapy, which has been found to lift mood, improve patients' interest in daily activities, and reduce aggressiveness and resistance to care. Music can be therapeutic at an outdoor concert, in a car, at home, and in any number of nonclinical settings. Singing to music or playing music also seem to have therapeutic benefits.

Other Therapeutic Activities

Early- and middle-stage Alzheimer's impairs cognition, but does not eliminate the need to engage in meaningful activity, move about as freely as possible, and interact with the rest of the world. Walking a dog, attending a religious service, or planting a garden can help make someone with dementia feel he is a person, not just someone suffering from a disease.

Pet Therapy

Dogs, cats, and other domestic pets can provide companionship and comfort to older people and may help lower stress and anxiety in people with Alzheimer's. Groups like the ASPCA train people-pet pairs, and people with early or mild AD who would benefit from animal companionship might consider going through the training. which may be suitable for someone with early or mild AD.

Essential

Songs and prayers tend to remain in memory long after Alzheimer's takes its toll. Try praying, singing songs or hymns, or reading spiritual passages with your loved one. He may not be able to talk about dinner or play checkers, but repeating a familiar prayer with you or sharing it with others can be a source of comfort.

More and more nursing homes and assisted living facilities are welcoming therapy dog visitors. The occasional canine presence seems to calm agitated patients and can also promote social interaction among people with Alzheimer's disease.

Pet therapy doesn't have to involve one-on-one contact with animals. Bird watching and looking at an in-home aquarium can be therapeutic as well, particularly for people in later stages of the disease.

Spiritual and Emotional Sustenance

Spirituality, faith, and religious rituals can help sustain people in sickness as well as in health and can be important for overall well-being. AD experts encourage family and caregivers to help people with dementia continue observing religious practices and traditions.

Taking someone with Alzheimer's to religious services isn't always easy. Some places of worship have special rooms designed for parents with noisy children, and those can also be used for someone with AD who becomes disruptive. You might look into religious services at a nearby senior center, where other worshippers may be suffering from dementia too. You can also try going to early morning services or visiting church or temple between regular services.

Spirituality can help both you and your loved one cope with the day-to-day difficulties of Alzheimer's disease.

Therapeutic Garden

Therapeutic gardens designed to help ailing people connect with nature are sprouting up at many health and rehabilitation facilities. Spending time in a pleasant outdoor setting can help reduce stress, lower blood pressure, and lift mood. Watching a sunset, listening to birds, or smelling fragrant trees and flowers can keep your loved one connected with the world around her. A safe, secure garden can be a place she enjoys and can allow her to continue activities she has done throughout her life. Gardening can also be a source of comfort and relaxation to caregivers and other family members who are spending time with someone with AD.

CHAPTER 18

Caring for the Person with Alzheimer's—and Yourself

E ach year, an estimated 44 million American caregivers provide $257 billion worth of care to their family members and friends. Few are trained—physically or emotionally—to take on roles traditionally performed by nurses and social workers caring for someone with a chronic illness. Physicians sometimes call family caregivers hidden patients because so many neglect their own health and well-being while taking care of others. Caregiving for Alzheimer's is particularly difficult, and it is critical to tap into the resources and get the support you need.

The Caregivers

Family caregivers do the shopping, make the meals, care for the household, pay the bills, keep track of appointments, and arrange transportation to and from medical visits. They nurse, bathe, feed, and console their loved ones.

In the United States, 65 percent of elders who need long-term care rely exclusively on family and friends to provide that assistance, according to the U.S. Administration on Aging. An additional 30 percent rely on family care supplemented with paid assistance.

Though more men are becoming involved in what some social scientists call informal assistance, several studies show that women are the primary caregivers for spouses, parents, parents-in-law, friends, and neighbors. Many are elders themselves, struggling with their own age-related disabilities and ailments. Most are middle-aged women, members of the so-called sandwich generation, who juggle caregiving with paying jobs and their own families' needs.

 Fact

> The typical American caregiver is a 46-year-old employed female baby boomer with some college education who works full- or part-time and spends more than twenty hours a week caring for her mother, who lives nearby. She balances family, work, and caregiving duties for an average of 4.3 years, according to a study by the National Alliance for Caregiving and AARP.

Caring for the Caregiver: The Basics

Caregivers are less likely to take care of themselves than are most other people, cautions the U.S. Department of Health and Human Services Administration on Aging. That puts them at greater risk for infectious diseases (colds and flu) and for chronic illnesses (diabetes, heart problems, and cancer) than most people. Their risk of developing depression is twice that of the general population. Government health experts urge caregivers to care for themselves:

- Be wise—immunize. The Centers for Disease Control recommend that caregivers get one influenza vaccine each year and one tetanus booster every ten years.
- Don't neglect your health. Schedule a yearly checkup that includes recommended cancer screenings for people your age.
- Be sure to tell your doctor you are a caregiver.
- Tell your doctor if you feel depressed or nervous.
- Take some time each day to do something enjoyable for yourself. Read, listen to music, telephone friends, or exercise.

- Eat healthy foods and don't skip meals.
- Find and tap into caregiver resources in your community as soon as possible. You may not feel that you need these resources now, but it's helpful information to have on hand for the future.

The Extra Demands of AD Care

In 2006, U.S. Supreme Court Justice Sandra Day O'Connor retired early—and reluctantly—to care for her husband, John, who had Alzheimer's disease. In the years before she stepped down from the bench, the first female Supreme Court justice sometimes brought her husband to work with her because he could not be left alone, she said. "Many caregivers make similarly difficult decisions each and every day," O'Connor told a hearing of the U.S. Senate Special Committee on Aging in 2008. "Sadly, these life-changing decisions are simply part of caring for someone with Alzheimer's." Alzheimer's makes extraordinary demands on individuals and those who love them.

Fact

Approximately 70 percent of the 5 million Americans who currently have Alzheimer's disease live at home. Ten million family members and friends supervise their care, according to the Alzheimer's Association. Most people with Alzheimer's live at home or in the community until the very late stages of the disease.

Alzheimer's disease moves more slowly than other fatal illnesses, and many AD caregivers spend the better part of a decade—or more—helping an increasingly helpless person cope with the ravages of a brain-robbing illness.

In the early stages, your loved one may only need help shopping for groceries, preparing meals, and managing finances or legal affairs. As his symptoms worsen, he'll need more consistent attention and assistance simply to stay safe and secure. Most people with Alzheimer's eventually need assistance with all personal care, from bathing to using a toilet.

Alzheimer's changes how a person thinks, acts, and feels. That presents singular challenges, even in the early stages. If your loved one forgets what's being said from one minute to the next, a simple conversation about what's for lunch can become complicated and frustrating for both of you.

 Alert

Caring for a person with Alzheimer's is a marathon, not a sprint, warns the Alzheimer's Association. Marshal your resources and find every bit of assistance available to conserve your strength for this exhausting journey.

As someone with AD loses the basic skills and abilities he's taken for granted throughout his adult life, he may feel inept, confused, and helpless. That makes some people uncooperative and resistant to care. Some become belligerent. Unfortunately, some patients take out frustrations on their caretakers. Elderly people with Alzheimer's also tend to suffer from other serious medical conditions, such as diabetes and congestive heart failure, which can complicate the care they need.

Creating a Caregiving Team

"Caring for an older person at home requires a team of people with different skills and perspectives," advise physicians at the American Geriatrics Society. "Doctors, nurses, social workers, and clergy all make important, specialized contributions, but family members or friends give the day-to-day care."

Alzheimer's is not a onetime problem to address and resolve. It is a progressive and debilitating disease that makes changing, increasing demands over time. It is important that everyone involved understand the demands of Alzheimer's—and that each of you knows it is virtually impossible for a single family member to fulfill the day-to-day and long-term needs of someone with AD.

Establishing Responsibilities

If you are the primary caregiver, put together a candid summary of the diagnosis and appraisals from any professionals involved in your loved one's care. Use this information to explain the situation to your family and to make clear that everyone has to help.

Essential

Consider joining a support group. If there aren't any in your area or you are unable to get out to one, try an online support group, where you will no doubt find people familiar with just about every problem—and solutions to the problems—you encounter.

Call a meeting of all adults involved. Make a list of questions and issues that have to be covered. Try to have a family conference to reach a consensus on major concerns, such as legal guardianship or where your loved one should live. If it's impossible for everyone to get together in one place, line up a conference call. Make sure someone takes notes and summarizes points of agreement and decisions. E-mail everyone a copy of the summary.

Working Together

Alzheimer's is a devastating diagnosis, and each family member responds differently to the disease. Each has different circumstances that affect how much he can participate in caring for a loved one with AD.

In times of crisis, many families revert to childhood roles and perceptions about who's the good one, the responsible one, or the black sheep. Some families assume that the daughters are more responsible than the sons for caring for parents who are ill.

Fact

It's important to recognize that everyone's role changes with Alzheimer's. The person with the disease can no longer perform his lifelong roles—as father, breadwinner, family vacation planner, or cook, for example. To function effectively, you and your family will probably have to rethink and revise your roles and responsibilities.

Counselors suggest families try a divide-and-conquer approach to dealing with AD care. Talk over each of your skills, strengths, and life situations. Discuss the best way for each person to contribute. A sibling who lives far away can't be intimately involved but may be able to research clinical trials, investigate housing options, or handle financial matters. A single parent who's employed part-time probably can't commit as much money as her high-powered executive sister. But either or both might be able to schedule weekend visits or vacations during which they care for their loved one and give the main provider a break.

THE VALUE OF A SUPPORT GROUP

Some older people—and a good number who are younger—think of support groups as group therapy sessions where people unload dark, painful, and devastating secrets about themselves or their loved ones. Or they imagine confrontational intervention sessions in which members encounter someone (usually a family member), who breaks down and confesses to ineptitude or bad behavior. Why, they ask, would I spend what little time I have talking to strangers in a charged, invasive, and odd environment?

Not knowing what to expect, not wanting to talk to strangers, and feeling that you should be able to handle a loved one's illness on your own are common reasons people shy away from support groups. Other reasons are being too busy, too tired, or too indispensable because no one else can take over at home for a couple of hours.

If you think you or someone you care about could use a little advice from people who are going through similar experiences, try to point out that support groups are generally informal meetings in which people talk about shared problems and solutions. Everyone has problems and solutions of their own. No one is required to share their feelings or cry. Though sharing frustration and sadness is part of many groups, so is laughter.

Women tend not to consider the importance of taking care of themselves when they're caring for someone with AD, experts say. But some may try a support group session if they think it will help them learn to take better care of their loved ones, and, in the course of doing that, do something for themselves.

If you think someone would benefit from a support group, do a little research and find different options in your area. The Alzheimer's Association or a nearby Area Agency on Aging can suggest some if your physicians don't know of any. Volunteer or arrange for someone to cover for the caregiver while she attends the session.

Common Sources of Family Conflict

When someone you love is suffering from Alzheimer's, your entire family lives with ongoing stress and grief, which can cause—and exacerbate—disagreements and conflicts.

It is not uncommon for a devoted spouse or adult child to deny the seriousness or extent of AD, therapists say. Sometimes, an overly protective spouse insists the patient's symptoms aren't all that bad, that others are overreacting, and that she can meet any of the loved one's needs. In other cases, an adult child who lives out of town and doesn't see the patient regularly maintains that his parent is perfectly safe living alone and that the patient's doctor and caregivers are alarmist or inept. Denial can manifest itself in unrealistic hopes that certain treatments or interventions will cure someone with Alzheimer's.

Refusing to recognize the extent of a loved one's illness and what it takes to keep a dementia patient safe and comfortable can stir up feelings of guilt and resentment among those with a more realistic grasp of the circumstances and can stand in the way of medical necessity and ancillary care. If conflicts arise in your family, consult a trusted friend, counselor, or clergy member to speak with everyone involved. You can also seek help from someone who specializes in dementia and geriatric care.

Fact

Learn as much as you can about the support services that are available in your community. These might range from senior centers and respite care to adult day care centers. Visiting nurses and other professional health service providers can help home caregivers with diet and nutrition as well as personal care issues, including incontinence and personal hygiene.

With the ranks of family caregivers growing by the day, you will probably be able to find someone who has encountered and resolved every problem you face. Tap into that expertise, be it in your immediate family circle, in your community, or online.

CHANGING FAMILY ROLES

"When I moved in with my mother, I knew we were changing roles. I was becoming the mother while she became the child," says Alice, 62, who was the primary caregiver for a mother with Alzheimer's for seven years.

What she didn't know was that other family roles would change. To Alice's surprise, she says, "My sisters expected me to be the mom and take care of Mom at the same time."

Like many people with AD, Alice's mother managed at first to live on her own with help from Alice. "For a couple of years before I moved in, I paid the bills, took her to the doctor, the hairdresser, her bingo games, the grandkids' birthday parties, that sort of thing," she recalls. "But then it got to the point where she couldn't do her own cooking or cleaning, and then she really wasn't safe. I quit my job and moved in with her. That was the only way we could keep her at home."

Alice's sisters, who lived nearby, expected her to take on their mother's lifelong roles, such as organizing family get-togethers and sitting in the front row at sports games, concerts, and plays. "They expected me, like Mom, to be there when they needed to drop off a sick kid, too," she recalls. "Like a lot of women her age, my mother didn't have a career. But she did a lot of work no one really noticed, because it always got done!

"There was absolutely no way I could play her role and mine as the live-in caretaker," Alice said. A friend urged Alice to write down every job and task involved in caring for her increasingly incapacitated mother.

The list covered a large sheet of paper. It included Alice's unpaid jobs as her mother's driver, cook, gardener, and personal aide; her financial, medical, legal and familial responsibilities; and the large and growing number of tasks of daily living—from bathing and grooming to eating—her mother could no longer accomplish by herself.

243

"It made me see that my role and my mother's role were both full-time jobs—and that I couldn't do both," said Alice. "And it gave me something specific to show my sisters that I needed help."

Becoming the Primary Caregiver

Twenty-five percent of family caregivers who take care of someone with Alzheimer's disease end up visiting an emergency room or checking into a hospital themselves every six months, according to an Indiana University study published in the November 2008 issue of the *Journal of General Internal Medicine*. Researchers attribute the incidents to the difficulty of coping with the ever-increasing physical demands and behavioral challenges of people with Alzheimer's.

Living with Grief

Many caregivers say the hardest part of caring for someone with dementia is the emotional impact of caring for someone who is "there but not there" or "slipping away." AD caregivers live through a slow, steady loss of a companion and source of support. Many AD caregivers experience what psychologists call anticipatory grief— the pain of losing someone who is terminally ill but hasn't yet died.

Alert

Try to avoid communicating only during crises such as a diagnosis or episodes like wandering. Use e-mail, form a family group on Facebook or another social networking site, or arrange occasional conference calls to communicate with one another about everyone's concerns and needs.

Caregivers may also live with ambiguous loss, a term psychologists use to describe the absence of someone who is alive but no longer socially, intellectually, or emotionally present. They grieve the loss of a spouse or parent who can no longer perform that role.

Many caregivers feel guilty about their particular, prolonged feelings of grief. Finding a support group or a confidant can help you cope with the feelings.

When You Can't Do It Alone

People who take on the job of caring for someone with dementia tend to be dedicated, independent, and resourceful, yet many are reluctant to ask for help. Some see doing so as an acknowledgment of failure. Others are so burdened with responsibilities and tasks that they don't know how or where to begin responding to people who say, "Call me if you need me" or "What can I do for you?"

Fact

Caregivers who take advantage of support groups, adult day care, and respite care services keep their Alzheimer's patient at home longer than those who do not, according to the American Geriatrics Society. They also tend to feel healthier and find caregiving more rewarding than those who do not use support services.

But as AD progresses, most patients require constant supervision and assistance with nearly every activity. Caregivers often find they are consumed with round-the-clock duties and can't keep up with basic at-home needs, like grocery shopping, laundry, and cleaning. Some let everything go.

Finding Professional Help

Try to identify what kind of help you most need. Do you need a daily break? Would you and your loved one benefit from being apart for a few hours? If your loved one is homebound, do you need a nurse to clean and bandage wounds and monitor equipment?

Would hiring a homecare aide to help your loved one get showered and dressed better suit your needs? Or should you consider hiring a companion/homemaker who can fill in for you for a few hours at a time?

GETTING HELP

Here are some tips for hiring in-home caregiver help.

1. Start looking long before you think you need help—even if you think you'll never need it.
2. Whether you hire someone through an agency or on your own, remember: You are an employer and she is an employee. Don't hire help solely based on cost. Some hospitals distribute lists of agencies and home care workers, and they tend to highlight the cheapest ones. This is not a place to cut corners.
3. Ask anyone who interviews for the job to bring a resume or written work history, personal identification (proof of name, address, date of birth), and references and contact information for two previous employers. Find out how much experience she has had working with people with dementia. Talk about the challenges of the job.
4. Trust your instincts. If you feel uncomfortable with something about the person during the interview process, don't hire her.
5. Write a job contract that clearly describes the job duties, days and hours to be worked, and pay rate, including when and in what form of currency the employee will be paid. If you hire someone who isn't referred by an agency, she is considered an independent contractor and you are obligated to report her earnings to the IRS. You may be responsible for paying taxes, so check with the IRS for forms and directions. The job contract should

stipulate a hire date, trial period, and termination policy; holiday, vacation and sick policy; and a contingency plan that covers your needs if the employee informs you on short notice that she can't come to work.

6. Be clear about your expectations and try to keep the relationship professional. You may become very fond of a homecare worker, but limits have to be set. Just because someone does a good job doesn't mean she makes the rules. Be clear from the outset that you want the worker to feel free to voice any complaints to you, and that you have the same right to voice your concerns.

7. Homecare workers are often eager to help but don't know what your loved one was like before she was ill. You can help fill in the gaps, which will likely improve her understanding and their time together.

8. Don't expect the homecare worker to handle important communications with doctors, lawyers, or other professionals. Don't share financial information with homecare workers. Keep records and accounts of all financial transactions; ask for receipts if she spends money you have given her on your behalf.

9. Keep the lines of communication open, and don't lose perspective. Don't be afraid to make a change if you feel there is friction. The best homecare workers are able to be honest without being defensive.

Adapted from an article by Steven Schwartzman, director of Elder Care New York, on eldercare.com.

You might also consider respite care. Respite care is designed to give you, the caregiver, a break. It includes adult day care programs, in-home help, and short nursing home stays. Adult day care programs range from all-day to occasional care at most senior and some community centers. Short-term respite care is available at many nursing homes or assisted-living facilities, which offer spare beds for short-term respite stays.

Question

What can I do if I feel torn by the realities of caring for someone with AD?
Many caregivers worry that their lives will be consumed by caring for their loved one. They may feel guilty for wanting their responsibilities to end because it will mean the death of a loved one. Try thinking "I am both a caregiver and a person with my own needs" or "I wish both that it was over—and that my loved one could keep on living."

A few organizations, such as the Family Caregiver's Alliance in California, offer weekend camps for people with cognitive impairment. Your best bet for finding programs near you is to do an online search for overnight senior respite care or eldercare in your town. If that isn't available, family members, friends, or others caring for sick people can fill in for you at home for short periods of time.

Informal Support: Asking Others for Help

Despite the fact that family caregivers are drowning in responsibility or are really confused about what the next step ought to be, they often reject offers of help. Recognize that asking for help is a sign of strength, not weakness. It means you truly have a grasp on your situation and have come up with a proactive problem-solving approach to making things easier and better. Take a breath and acknowledge that having some help will make a real difference in your loved one's quality of life—and yours as well.

THE IMPACT OF CAREGIVING ON A PARTNER OR SPOUSE

If you are caring for a parent with Alzheimer's, your duties and demands are almost certain to put significant pressure on your relationship with your partner or spouse, according to a survey conducted by Caring.com, the online eldercare resource center.

Eighty percent of the 300 family caregivers who responded to the survey said that caring for an older relative had put a strain on their relationship or marriage. "Decreased time together, lack of opportunity for consistent communication, resentment of the needy parent, shift in the use of financial resources, increased fatigue and stress all increase the strain on a marriage," the survey concluded.

Couples were most likely to feel undue strain if the caregiver was holding down a paid job, if they were providing financial assistance to an aging relative, or if the elder person lived in their home. Nine out of ten respondents said caregiving caused them to spend more time apart from their spouse, and nearly half said that was causing them to drift apart. Forty-six percent of those surveyed said that caregiving had a negative impact on their romantic relationship with their significant other, and 34 percent said it had a negative impact on their sexual relationship.

However, 20 percent of respondents said caregiving caused no strain on their primary relationship. Indeed, some said it had brought them closer together. "My husband knows that my mother won't be here forever and tells me to do what I feel like I have to do, and I love him dearly for this," one respondent said.

Prioritize

Caregiving, like any job, is made up of many individual tasks, not all of which are of the same importance. Some tasks are easy; others require some skill and fortitude. The challenge is to know the difference. Think about and decide what help you need. Some—not all—duties and tasks are easier for you to do than to delegate to others. But paid professionals, family, or friends can handle some.

Create a list of your caregiving worries—such as what you'll do when Dad is home this summer along with the kids—and smaller tasks that need to be done in any given week. Group your tasks into categories that make sense to you.

This can help you think more rationally, prioritize your concerns, and recognize that getting help with some smaller tasks might lessen your stress. It can also give you ideas about what family members, friends, or community volunteers might be able to do to help.

HIRING A CAREGIVER

Once you bite the bullet and decide to hire a home caregiver or companion, get ready to bite down more, says Tom, a retired realtor who cares for his wife, Ellen. "Finding someone good who fits with your family situation is a big job," he says. "Finding someone who will stay is stupendous."

Tom hired four different companions for Ellen over a six-month period, and none lasted more than six weeks. "It wasn't that they weren't good. They were good to great," he laments. "But life is complicated—yours and theirs."

Ellen didn't like the first companion, and Tom suspects it was because she felt uncomfortable revealing her illness to a stranger for the first time. "My daughter said the first one would never work out, and I think she was right," he said.

He searched and found a "perfect" companion, who got along famously with Ellen for three weeks—until she was offered a job with overnight hours, at better pay. "The third person we hired loved us and we loved her," says Tom. "But her family moved an hour away, and the commute was too

long. She recommended a friend for the job, who was great."
But that companion had to leave in less than a week to take
care of her own ailing mother.

"You've got to realize this is very hard work," says Tom.
"The people who do it don't get paid much, and they have a
lot of demands on themselves. Life intervenes."

Avoid Caregiver Burnout

Caregiver burnout is one of the main reasons people with Alzheimer's are placed in nursing homes, specialists say. "Caregiving for a loved one can be one of the most stressful events you ever experience," according to Johns Hopkins University experts. AD caregivers are more likely than others to report that their own health is fair or poor. They are also more inclined to become socially isolated and to become embroiled in family disagreements. The doctors urge caregivers to pay attention to both physical and emotional health, and to watch out for these common signs of caregiver stress:

❏ Feeling sad or moody
❏ Crying more often than usual
❏ Having low energy levels
❏ Feeling trapped
❏ Feeling as if you don't have any time to yourself
❏ Experiencing trouble sleeping or not wanting to get out of
   bed in the morning
❏ Overeating or eating too little
❏ Seeing friends or relatives less often
❏ Losing interest in people and things you enjoy
❏ Feeling angry with the person you are caring for or at other
   people or situations

The key to overcoming burnout is to stay in touch with the people and activities you enjoy—even if you sometimes feel too exhausted or overwhelmed to get in touch or go out. Talk to your family and friends and take up their offers to help. Don't hesitate to consult a doctor about your feelings.

Look for help in your community. You may start by asking your church or synagogue if they provide services or have volunteers who can help you. You can also ask for help from support organizations.

Fact

If you are a primary caregiver, you may not think anyone else can anticipate or solve your loved one's physical and emotional problems. But it's important to think of yourself as a team member and work cooperatively with others to cope with the escalating demands of caregiving. Otherwise, you are jeopardizing your health and well-being and your loved one's care.

Finally, remember the positive. Caring for someone with Alzheimer's disease can be challenging and frustrating, but you and your loved one will still laugh and enjoy life together. Cherish those moments.

CHAPTER 19

Living with Alzheimer's

You may think it's impossible to live well with AD. The diagnosis changes your life irrevocably. But it doesn't end it. The good news about Alzheimer's is that thousands of individuals have enjoyed many happy, productive years after their diagnosis. Their loved ones have sought and found treatments, techniques, and solutions that can help you not just survive Alzheimer's, but live securely and comfortably with people you most care about, doing things you enjoy.

How Bad Isn't It?

Most of what we know about people living with Alzheimer's is grim. Media reports show helpless patients and caregivers who can barely cope, all of them miserable and isolated. But most people with mild to moderate Alzheimer's still have the ability to enjoy life, according to an Alzheimer's Disease International (ADI) survey of 1,000 patients and caregivers in five countries.

Most among the more than 500 respondents with Alzheimer's said they enjoyed warm relationships with their caregivers. Most said they felt safe and supported at home. And more than 80 percent said they continued to "keep a social life with their family and friends" and felt "well-respected by family members."

The 2007 survey did not ignore the difficulties of living with Alzheimer's disease. A majority of caregivers, for example, said "caring for someone with AD is burdensome."

Nevertheless, more than 70 percent reported that taking care of someone with Alzheimer's helped them "appreciate what's really important" in life, that it's a way of repaying some of the love and care they received in the past. And more than half called the work "rewarding."

An Alzheimer's Bill of Rights

Bioethicist Nancy Dubler is believed to be the first person to propose a Bill of Rights for Alzheimer's patients and their families. The principles, which many have adapted and modified, are summarized here. As someone living with Alzheimer's, you have the right:

❏ To the most thorough and accurate diagnosis and treatment available

❏ To be informed about your diagnosis and results of all tests

❏ To start treatment before losing additional functions, and to receive appropriate, ongoing medical care

❏ To participate as long as possible in decisions about your present and future, including where you live and who provides your care

❏ To be productive in work and play as long as possible

❏ To be treated as an adult, not a child

❏ To express your feelings and be taken seriously

❏ To live in a safe, structured, and predictable environment

❏ To enjoy meaningful activities each day

❏ To exercise as appropriate

❏ To be out-of-doors on a regular basis

❏ To have physical contact

❏ To be cared for in proximity to people who know your life story, and who respect your cultural and religious traditions

❏ To be cared for by individuals well trained in dementia care

If you feel your needs and wishes are overlooked, talk to a counselor or other people with AD. Join a support group in your community or online.

Alzheimer's Is Not Your Entire Life

Caregiving involves enormous responsibilities, daily challenges, and a seemingly endless number of small duties and tasks that can wear down even the most patient providers. If all you do is deal with Alzheimer's, you're more likely to become isolated, stressed, and depressed.

 Alert

People with AD and those who care for them share a lot. Unfortunately, both tend to lose their sense of competence and self-esteem. Do things that will make both of you feel better. Get your hair cut. Give one another shoulder massages, or go for manicures.

Don't let Alzheimer's caregiving take up all your time, say mental health experts:

1. Interact and socialize with other people. Go to a meeting or class outside the home. When you're at home, spend time with your grandchildren or talk on the phone.
2. Do something that gives you a sense of accomplishment. Cook or bake something delicious. Choose a project and finish it. Set an exercise goal, such as getting in shape to run a race, and work to meet it. Help someone accomplish something.
3. Do at least one thing you enjoy. Watch a movie, walk outdoors, sing and dance along to your favorite CD, or work with plants.

CATHERINE'S STORY

Catherine thrived on being with people. Spending time with her children and grandchildren was her "lifeblood," she said. As she started to develop Alzheimer's symptoms, however, the family gatherings and dinners with friends she lived for left her frustrated and confused.

A trio of grandchildren home from college dropped by unannounced, assuming Gramma would be delighted. But to their surprise the visit distressed her—and them. Catherine had trouble telling her grandsons apart, and couldn't follow their conversation.

People with Alzheimer's need people. They also need predictability and quiet, experienced caregivers say. The following strategies may help you meet both needs.

- **Eat in.** Restaurants are loud, distracting, and confusing to many people with dementia. Order from a favorite restaurant and enjoy the meal in her home.
- **Visit at the time of day that's best for your loved one.** Check with her caregiver beforehand.
- **Visit alone or with one other person when possible.** People with AD do better one-on-one.
- **Even if you're there to lift her spirits, try to be calm and quiet.** When you arrive, try to establish eye contact. Call her by her name and remind her who you are. She may or may not recognize you when you first arrive.
- **Keep the conversation simple and in the present.** If we haven't seen someone in a while, it's normal to ask about what's happened since. ("How was your weekend?" "Did you get to see Mike when he was in town?") Try to remember that questions like these can be taxing for someone with memory problems. They might feel like a challenge or a test.

- **Avoid speaking loudly or as if you were talking to a child.**
- **Conversation is harder on some days than others.** Consider bringing along some photos, a video, or even a game you can share in case she isn't particularly talkative when you're there. You may not want or need it. But you may be pleased and relieved to have it on hand.

"Seniors should be encouraged to read, play board games, and go ballroom dancing," Dr. Joseph T. Coyle of Harvard Medical School wrote in a *New England Journal of Medicine* editorial, commenting on a twenty-one-year study of seniors ages seventy-five and older that compared different leisure activities with rates of dementia.

What Do You Do Every Day?

To someone with Alzheimer's, the world grows increasingly less familiar—and more fraught with uncertainties.

Question

The kids want to spend time with Grandma, but they're not sure what to do with her. Any ideas?
See the "101 Activities" suggestions on the Alzheimer's Association website *(www.alz.org/living_with_alzheimers_101_activities.asp)*. The site also has special information and activities for children and teenagers living with someone affected by Alzheimer's.

Do your best to maintain an environment that feels familiar, comfortable, and safe for your loved one. Concentrate on routines and plan his schedule so it includes activities he knows and enjoys. If he's a sports fan, be sure to turn on the game. If he's a lifelong churchgoer, try to take him to a service (or ask someone else to take him) once in a while.

Routines are essential. Schedule activities regularly, at the same time every day if possible, to enhance your loved one's sense of stability. Be cautious in planning activities that might demand skills and abilities he is losing or has lost. Be aware of physical limitations (lack of spatial orientation or coordination), and whether he can start an activity on his own. Alzheimer's can be unpredictable as well as demanding. Planning a schedule frees you from trying to figure out what to do from moment to moment.

A SAMPLE DAILY ROUTINE

Morning
Wash, brush teeth, get dressed
Prepare and eat breakfast
Discuss the newspaper or reminisce about old photos
Take a break, have some quiet time
Afternoon
Prepare and eat lunch, read mail, wash dishes
Listen to music or do a crossword puzzle
Take a walk
Evening
Prepare and eat dinner
Play cards, watch a movie, or give a massage
Take a bath, get ready for bed

Source: *The Alzheimer's Association*

If your loved one responds well to an activity, do it over and over again. Research studies show that the following activities are therapeutic for people with AD, and may reduce problem behavior:

❏ Playing music your loved one enjoys
❏ Interacting one-on-one
❏ Playing videotapes of family members
❏ Walking and gentle exercise
❏ Pet therapy

Physical activity can help prevent muscle weakness and health complications that develop in people who are sedentary. Getting exercise encourages a normal day-and-night routine, which may help boost your loved one's mood. While exercise won't stop the progression of AD, it can provide emotional satisfaction and a feeling of accomplishment.

Remember to Enjoy

The best activities have a purpose; they let someone with AD know she is wanted or needed. But they should focus on enjoyment, not achievement.

Craft activities are good for promoting eye-hand coordination, and they might provide some pleasure and fun. Music is therapeutic, but it's also enjoyable for most people.

The creative arts are unstructured, uninhibited, and unexpected—just as AD can be on the good days. Even if your loved one has never been artsy, consider helping her try storytelling (or blogging), dancing, or singing. Visit Don Moyer's blog for people with memory loss, Dancing Away Memory Blues (*http:// dancing-away-memory-blues.blogspot.com*) for a treasure trove of suggestions.

Getting the Help You Need at Home and Online

Every bit of help you can get as an Alzheimer's caregiver gives you more energy to spend with your loved one.

How Can I/You/They Help?

Caregiving works best if you have a network of family and friends you can count on for help and support.

Check out Lotsa Helping Hands (*www.lotsahelpinghands .com/home*), a free online community whose website helps organize family members, friends, neighbors, and colleagues during times of need.

Use the Internet

Broadband Internet access is an invaluable resource for people living with AD. It can connect you with friends, family, and services that vastly improve your quality of life. It offers information and instruction condensed in fact and tip sheets that can help you understand and meet the medical, legal, financial, and practical challenges that are part and parcel of Alzheimer's.

However, make sure you get your information from a reputable source. There are websites that tout miracle cures without any information to back up their claims.

The sheer volume of health information online—and its wildly uneven quality—makes sorting the wheat from chaff difficult, according to Susannah Fox of Pew Internet and American Life Project. Most e-patients start with search engines like Google or Yahoo, which turn up thousands of websites, ranked according to the appearance of key words. This doesn't necessarily lead to reliable information.

Alert

If you type Aricept or Namenda into the Google search box, the first results displayed will be the websites of the pharmaceutical companies who manufacture the drugs. Many of these large, slick sites are packed with health information, some of which is authoritative and useful. But corporate websites are marketing tools designed to sell products. Do not rely on them as independent sources of information.

To distinguish science from pseudoscience and snake oil, follow these suggestions, adapted from the Medical Library Association and MayoClinic.com guidelines, which can help you get to the most accurate, comprehensive, and user-friendly health sites.

1. **Consider the source.** Who sponsors the site and produces its material? Is it a government health agency site (.gov), an association or nonprofit (.org), or someone with a blog and strong opinions about Alzheimer's care and treatment? Click the "About" or "About us" links on the home page to find out the site sponsor. Websites created by major medical centers, universities, and government agencies are the most credible.

2. **Is the site trying to sell you something?** Some dot-com sites support excellent content, but they may also come with advertising, which may be posted by a reputable health care provider. If the site features content about that advertiser, watch out. Stay away from sites that don't distinguish clearly between factual evidence and advertisements. Be wary, too, of commercial sites or personal testimonials that promote a single, simple solution or incredible cure.

3. **When was the page last updated?** Check the bottom of the page. This is particularly important as new health and science studies and evidence emerges that can contradict what a site published just last year. Pay attention to whether articles are updated.

Caregiver Bookmarks

Appendix B lists many caregiver resources. Bookmark these essential websites now so that you will have access to reliable, accessible information on health and medicine, caregiving, and how best to link to sources and resources you need.

Communicating with Alzheimer's

In the middle stages of Alzheimer's, many people withdraw from family, friends, and social activities. A family get-together or class reunion your mother might have loved a year or two earlier is now bewildering and distressing. She can't remember names, the word for the vehicle she arrived in, or the outer garment she has checked at the restaurant. While she recognizes old friends and remembers the wonderful times they had together, she can't follow what they're saying now. To make matters worse, she's confounded by the sequence of courses at lunch. That is upsetting and confusing, says Coach Frank Broyles.

Dealing with Withdrawal

Normally gregarious people may withdraw at this stage because they are losing their ability to grasp what people around them are saying. "It is getting hard for her to shut out noises around her. She can't focus on what is being said," Broyles says. He suggests limiting the number of people your loved one interacts with in social situations and at home. "Have guests talk with her away from the crowd and noise," he suggests. "If she gets upset, move to a quiet area with her until she becomes calm."

Joanne Koenig Coste, author of *Learning to Speak Alzheimer's*, maintains that "people with Alzheimer's stop speaking not because they lose their ability to understand and communicate, but because they're afraid of being wrong."

People with AD are responding to fear and a "feeling that they're not worth anything anymore," says Coste. "We stop including the person when it seems like they can no longer give us any information that is useful to us. That doesn't matter! They need to be included. Ask the person what he wants for supper even if you know the answer is going to be 'Whatever you're making.' So what! You've included him and made him feel like he's still worth something."

Your loved one may also withdraw because the world around her—the one her loved ones live in—is no longer familiar.

"It makes them very frustrated, and logically so," Coste said in an interview with Caring.com. "Wouldn't it be frustrating to us if somebody was insisting that it's 2012 when we know it's 2008? Well, that's how they feel, and that's why they often stop talking. If they're going to make a mistake every time they talk, they're not going to talk."

Really Listen

When someone gets distressed because she can't communicate, be patient and calm. "Stop what you are doing. Really listen to what she is trying to say. Think about the feelings behind the words she is trying to say. Look at what her body is trying to tell you. If she looks upset or angry, then ask her if she is," Broyles advises. "Treat her with dignity and respect."

Essential

Try reassuring an anxious person with gentle, strategic touch. Touch can convey companionship, safety, and reassurance. When your loved one is confused, maintain some physical contact with her. Hold her hand or arm. This can also help orient a confused or sight-impaired person.

"I want to go home" is the most common lament of people with Alzheimer's, who may sometimes want to go home when they're in their own house. In this situation, Coste says that desire can be translated as "'I want you to hug me and make me feel at home, that I'm in a place where I'm secure.' And that's what we need to do."

The Middle to Late Stages of Alzheimer's

Middle to late-stage Alzheimer's is sometimes called "the long goodbye." The disease causes volatile emotions, and those may lead to mood swings, crying, agitation, and outbursts doctors call catastrophic reactions: shouting, cursing, or even hitting others.

People with AD have difficulty comprehending what others say or do, and this may spur agitation, anger, and delusions (accusing a spouse of infidelity, talking to imaginary people, thinking a reflection in a mirror is a stranger). As Alzheimer's progresses, your loved one may engage in obsessive behavior, such as cleaning one object over and over or removing and replacing the contents of a drawer. She may pace, wring her hands, or ask the same question repeatedly.

Many people with AD sleep fitfully. They may awaken at night with hallucinations, feeling frightened and disoriented and unable to go back to sleep. That can trigger nighttime wandering.

Nearing the End

Contrary to what many people think—and what you may wish—people with Alzheimer's don't succumb peacefully to their disease. The final, most debilitating stage of Alzheimer's can last two to three years. During that time, your loved one will lose awareness of her surroundings and her ability to speak. She may not recognize you and others. She will probably lose control of her bladder and bowels. She will grow dependent on others to help her walk, sit up, and eventually swallow.

Bedridden, she will most likely need round-the-clock, hands-on care. She may develop severe joint pain and stiffness. She will be prone to pneumonia, urinary tract infections, dehydration, malnutrition, and bedsores. These conditions are commonly listed as causes of death among people with AD.

End-of-Life Medical Care

Medical care for people with advanced Alzheimer's should concentrate on daily care and comfort, not treatments that will cure illness or prolong life, Alzheimer's and geriatric specialists say. Make sure copies of advance medical directives are in your loved one's medical chart so staff at a hospital or nursing home will know what is and isn't to be done in medical emergencies.

The Alzheimer's Association's ethics advisory panel advises against using life-extending technologies and treatments. In the panel's opinion, measures that "prolong life in the advanced stage of Alzheimer's result in unnecessary suffering for people who could otherwise reach the end of life in relative comfort and peace."

You and your family may want to consider hospice care, which focuses entirely on pain management and comfort care, for your loved one. Typically, hospices care for people who have less than six months to live. Because it can be so difficult to predict how long a person with end-stage Alzheimer's will live, getting approved for hospice care can sometimes be a challenge. The National Hospice and Palliative Care Organization (*www.nhpco.org*) has published guidelines to help doctors determine when hospice is appropriate for people with Alzheimer's disease.

As the end approaches, follow this advice from Coach Broyles: "While your loved one may not know who you are, she still has feelings. Her need for love and touch has never been greater than it is now. She can still feel scared, rejected, lonely or sad." Now is a time to hold her, talk to her, stroke her gently, and show your love and support.

Glossary

Acetylcholine
A neurotransmitter crucial to memory and learning.

Age-associated memory impairment
Normal forgetfulness that increases with age.

Activities of daily living (ADLs)
Eating, bathing, grooming, dressing, and going to the toilet.

Acute care
Acute care is a medical setting such as a hospital, intensive care unit, or emergency department that provides short-term, temporary care.

Adult day care
A safe, supervised daytime program for disabled adults that offers basic health care, activities, and opportunities for people to socialize. Most centers are community based and open during weekday business hours; some programs also run during the evenings and on weekends.

Advance directive
A legal document outlining what kind of medical treatment you do and do not want if your life is in danger and you can't communicate. Advance directives include a living will, which details your wishes about medical treatments at the end of life, and a health care power of attorney, which lets you choose someone to make medical decisions for you.

Adverse reaction
An unwanted, adverse effect; side effect.

Amnesia (amnestic syndrome)
Severe memory loss that doesn't affect intelligence, general knowledge, awareness, attention span, judgment, personality, or identity.

Amyloid plaques
Dense deposits of beta-amyloid, pieces of damaged nerve cells, and other proteins found in the brains of people with Alzheimer's disease.

Antidepressant
A drug or intervention used to treat or prevent depression.

Antipsychotic
A medication believed to be effective in the treatment of psychosis. Sometimes called neuroleptic.

Anxiety

A feeling of apprehension and fear characterized by physical symptoms such as heart palpitations, sweating, and feelings of stress. Unlike passing periods of anxiety, anxiety disorders are chronic and serious medical illnesses that affect approximately 19 million American adults.

Aphasia

Partial or complete inability to use or understand language.

Apolipoprotein E (ApoE)

A gene found on chromosome 19 that codes for a protein that helps carry cholesterol in the bloodstream. The ApoE gene comes in several different forms. The E4 version of this gene is associated with an increased risk of Alzheimer's disease.

Approved drugs

Those approved by the Food and Drug Administration (FDA). The agency must approve a substance as a drug before it can be marketed.

Arm (of a study)

Any of the treatment groups in a randomized trial. Most randomized trials have two arms, but some have three or more.

Assistive device

Aids such as eyeglasses, a cane, a wheelchair, or a hearing aid.

Bed-bound or bed-fast

A person who is bed-bound cannot walk or get out of bed without help from another person or a mechanical lift.

Benzodiazepines

A class of drugs that act as tranquilizers and are commonly used in the treatment of anxiety. Benzodiazepines can cause drowsiness.

Beta-amyloid

A sticky, starch-like protein that is the main component of amyloid plaques.

Blind study

A research study in which participants don't know whether they are in an experimental or control group. In double-blind studies, neither participants nor researchers know who is receiving a treatment and who is getting placebo.

Bias

Point of view that prevents impartial judgment.

Cerebellum

A fist-sized structure located at the base of the brain beneath the cerebral cortex; it coordinates movement and balance.

Cerebral cortex

The wrinkled outer layer of gray matter that constitutes the "thinking" portion of the brain.

Cholinesterase inhibitors
Medications that slow the breakdown of acetylcholine, prescribed to treat Alzheimer's disease.

Chromosome
Microscopically visible carriers of the genetic material, composed of deoxyribonucleic acid (DNA) and proteins. Humans normally have 46 chromosomes.

Chronic care
Long-term care of individuals with long-standing, persistent diseases or conditions.

Circadian rhythm
The sleep/wake cycle.

Clinical
Pertaining to observation and treatment of human participants; distinguished from theoretical or basic science.

Cognitive
Refers to brain processes such as thinking, attention, perception, learning, memory, reasoning, problem solving, decision making, and planning. Cognitive processes are distinguished from emotional processes (feelings) and behavioral processes (actions).

Cohort
In epidemiology, a group of individuals with some characteristics in common.

Compassionate use
Providing experimental therapeutics to sick individuals prior

to final FDA approval of those drugs for use in humans. Compassionate use is usually invoked for acutely ill individuals who have no other treatment options.

Computed tomography (CT)
An imaging technology that uses x-rays to create a two-dimensional image of the brain or other parts of the body.

Contraindication
A specific circumstance in which use of certain treatments could be harmful.

Creutzfeldt-Jakob disease (CJD)
A rare, fatal brain disorder that causes a rapid, progressive dementia; sometimes mistaken for Alzheimer's disease.

Declarative memory
Recalling newly learned information about people, places, and things.

Dementia
Significant loss of memory and other intellectual abilities such as attentiveness that is severe enough to interfere with normal daily functioning.

DNA
Deoxyribonucleic acid. One of two types of molecules that encode genetic information. (The other is RNA, which carries DNA's message from the cell nucleus to the cytoplasm.)

Dopamine

Neurotransmitter linked to pleasure, movement, and sexual desire. A dopamine deficiency in certain areas of the brain results in Parkinson's disease.

Dose-ranging study

A clinical trial in which two or more doses of an agent (such as a drug) are tested against each other to determine which dose works best and is least harmful.

Double-blind study

A research study in which neither the participants nor the study staff know which participants are receiving the experimental treatment and which are getting either a standard treatment or a placebo.

Double-masked study

A double-blind study.

Durable power of attorney

A legal form that names someone (sometimes called an agent) to act as your substitute. "Durable" means that the agent can act for you once you are disabled or incapacitated. (See Power of Attorney.)

Dementia with Lewy bodies (Lewy body dementia)

A type of dementia characterized early in the disease by impaired executive function, disorientation, falls, and hallucinations, as well as signs of Parkinsonism.

Drug-drug interaction

A modification of the effect of a drug when administered with another drug. The effect may increase or decrease the effectiveness of either substance, or induce an adverse effect that is not normally associated with either drug.

Efficacy

The maximum ability of a drug or treatment to produce a result regardless of dosage. A drug passes efficacy trials if it is effective at the dose tested and against the illness for which it is prescribed. In the procedure mandated by the FDA, Phase II clinical trials gauge efficacy, and Phase III trials confirm it.

Elder law attorney

An attorney who handles estate planning, conservatorships, and other issues most common among older adults.

Empirical

Based on observed information or data, not on a theory.

Enzymes

Complex protein (or protein-based molecule) that speeds up a chemical reaction in a living organism.

Epidemiology

Study of populations in order to determine the frequency and distribution of disease and measure risks. An epidemiological study is a population-based research study.

Executive function

The ability to carry out familiar tasks, such as getting dressed or balancing a checkbook. Executive functioning includes the ability to plan projects, formulate goals and objectives, prioritize, apply self-discipline, and remember steps involved in complex tasks.

Alzheimer's disease gradually deteriorates executive functioning, making it increasingly difficult to carry out daily tasks and live independently. Because it's hard to assess during a medical visit, health professionals usually rely on reports from the caregiver and the person with Alzheimer's to evaluate executive functioning.

Financial planner

Helps client manage their financial resources.

Free radicals

A particularly reactive atom or group of atoms that has at least one unpaired electron and is therefore unstable. In animal tissues, free radicals can damage cells, proteins, and DNA by altering their chemical structure. Free radicals are believed to accelerate the progression of cancer, cardiovascular disease, and age-related diseases.

Frontotemporal dementia

A spectrum of brain disorders that attack the frontal and temporal lobes, impairing motivation, judgment, personality, language, and social awareness. People with this dementia often engage in rash, antisocial behavior and are seldom aware they have lost any mental function.

Functional impairment

Inability to dress, use the toilet, eat, bathe, or walk without help.

Gene

The basic biological unit of heredity. A segment of deoxyribonucleic acid (DNA) needed to contribute to a function.

Geriatric care manager

In most cases, a licensed nursing or social work professional who specializes in geriatrics and who helps evaluate and assess elders' needs and coordinate care through community resources. Can function as a "professional relative" or surrogate to interact with agencies like Medicaid, help families identify and meet needs, and mediate difficult family discussions.

Gray matter

The area of the brain, gray in appearance, that contains cell bodies (in contrast to white matter, which contains the nerve fibers that extend from the cell bodies).

Hallucinations

A sensory experience that seems real to the person experiencing it, though it is not actually happening. The most common hallucinations are visual (seeing something that isn't really there) and auditory (hearing something that isn't really there).

Hippocampus
A small structure in the brain that plays a major role in emotion and memory.

Hospice
Facility or program dedicated to the care and comfort of terminally ill people and their families.

Huntington's disease
A rare, hereditary disorder of the central nervous system characterized by uncontrollable movements and dementia. Also called Huntington's chorea.

Hypothesis
A supposition or an assumption advanced as a basis for reasoning or argument, or as a guide to experimental investigation.

Incontinence
An inability to control urination or defecation.

Inflammation
Bodily reaction to infection, irritation, or other injury, characterized by redness, warmth, swelling, and pain.

Interventions
In clinical trials, the primary interventions being studied, whether drug, gene transfer, vaccine, behavior, device, or procedure.

Investigational new drug
A new drug, antibiotic drug, or biological drug that is used in a clinical investigation. It also includes a biological product used in vitro for diagnostic purposes.

Lewy bodies
Abnormal structures found in cells throughout the brain in people who have Lewy body dementia as well as Parkinson's disease.

Long-term memory
Stores information learned recently and as long ago as early childhood.

Magnetic resonance imaging (MRI)
Radiology imaging technique that uses a powerful magnet, radio waves, and a computer, rather than x-rays, to produce images of internal structures of the body.

Medicaid
Medicaid is a government health program for low-income people.

Medicaid-certified
A Medicaid-certified facility can offer services to people who are on Medicaid.

Medicare
Medicare is a government health insurance program for people age 65 and older and for disabled people.

Medicare-certified
A Medicare-certified facility can offer services to people who are on Medicare.

Mini Mental State Examination (MMSE)
A short test, usually administered in a doctor's office, that measures basic skills such as short-term memory, long-term memory, writing, and speaking.

Mild cognitive impairment (MCI)
Forgetfulness that is worse than normal for one's age but is not associated with certain cognitive problems common in dementia, such as disorientation or confusion. The severity of MCI falls between that of age-associated memory impairment and early dementia.

Neurodegenerative
Relating to or characterized by degeneration of nervous tissue.

Neurofibrillary tangles
Deposits of the protein tau that accumulate inside nerve cells, making them unable to carry out normal function; found in the brains of people with Alzheimer's disease.

Neuron
Nerve cell.

Neurotransmitter
A specialized chemical that relays messages between nerve cells.

New drug application (NDA)
Application submitted by the manufacturer of a drug to the FDA after clinical trials have been completed for a license to market the drug for a specified indication.

Nonsteroidal anti-inflammatory drugs (NSAIDs)
One of a number of commonly prescribed medications for the inflammation of arthritis and other body tissues, such as in tendinitis and bursitis. Being tested for use in treating AD.

Neurotransmitter
Chemical messenger that transmits neurologic information from one cell to another across a synapse.

Off-label use
A drug prescribed for conditions other than those approved by the FDA.

Orphan drugs
FDA term for medications used to treat rare diseases and conditions. Pharmaceutical companies have few financial incentives to develop such drugs.

Parkinsonism
Symptoms of Parkinson's disease, such as tremors; rigid, stooped posture; and shuffling gait.

Parkinson's disease
A progressive neurological disease characterized by tremors, stooped posture, slow movement, poor balance, and shuffling gait.

Pick's disease

A form of frontotemporal dementia characterized by language difficulties, the inability to initiate a task or activity, problems with goal setting, personality changes, and loss of social skills. People with this disease are unaware they have lost any mental function.

Peer review

Review of a clinical trial by experts, chosen by the study sponsor, who evaluate the trial's scientific merit, participant safety, and ethical considerations.

Pharmacokinetics

The processes in a living organism of absorption, distribution, metabolism, and excretion of a drug or vaccine.

Prednisone

A steroid drug with powerful anti-inflammatory effects that is being tested as a treatment for Alzheimer's disease.

Power of attorney

Legal form that names someone to act as your substitute, but not if you are incapacitated.

PET scan

Positron emission tomography, a highly specialized imaging technique using short-lived radioactive substances. This technique produces three-dimensional colored images.

Placebo

Inactive pill, liquid, or powder that has no treatment value. Experimental treatments in clinical trials are compared with placebos to assess treatment effects.

Statistical significance

An outcome is statistically significant if it is unlikely that it occurred by chance.

Synapse

The point of connection usually between two nerve cells. More specifically, a specialized junction at which a nerve cell (a neuron) communicates with a target cell.

Tau

Protein that becomes toxic when it accumulates and twists into neurofibrillary tangles inside brain cells.

Respite care

Respite care provides temporary relief from caregiving tasks. Such care could include in-home assistance, a short nursing home stay, or adult day care.

Vascular dementia

Dementia resulting from impaired blood flow to the brain.

Visuospatial disturbance

A disturbance in the ability to correctly perceive the relationship between an object and the space around it or its relation to other objects or the self.

APPENDIX B

Resources

Housing Help

Assisted Living Federation of America (ALFA)

A national organization for professionally operated assisted living communities for older adults. Offers information for people interested in learning more about assisted living or finding a residence.

703-894-1805
www.alfa.org

SNAPforSeniors *www.snapforseniors.com*

Offers a free, searchable housing locator with 60,000 listings that comprise assisted living, residential care, nursing care and rehabilitation, continuing care retirement, and independent living facilities.

Government Programs and Assistance

Alzheimer's Disease Education and Referral Center (ADEAR)

Part of the NIH's National Institute on Aging (NIA), ADEAR offers comprehensive information and publications on diagnosis, treatment, patient care, caregiver needs, long-term care, research, and more. Searchable online database.

P.O. Box 8250
Silver Spring, MD 20907-8257
800-438-4380
www.alzheimers.nia.nih.gov

Area Agency on Aging (AAA)

AAAs are part of a nationwide network of local elder service providers (such as senior centers, affordable housing programs, and eldercare programs) that offer a wide variety of in-home services, including:

- Meals On Wheels
- Homemaking (help with tasks such as grocery shopping and housekeeping)
- Home repair, yard, and other household services
- Personal care providers, who assist with bathing and feeding
- Respite care, to provide a short break for caregivers

You can find AAAs through ElderCare Locator.

Eldercare Locator *www.govbenefits.gov*

Need meals, home care, transportation, caregiver training? Contact Eldercare Locator, a free, nationwide directory assistance service that helps older people and their caregivers find local support and resources.

800-677-1116
www.eldercare.gov

Govbenefits.gov

An online tool that helps you determine eligibility for a variety of government programs and assistances.

Medicare.gov

Central source with links to all Medicare coverage and services. Information on insurance, prescription drugs, health costs. Tools such as Nursing Home Compare provide detailed information about the past performance of every Medicare and Medicaid-certified nursing home in the country. A special resource for caregivers' questions is available online at *www.medicare.gov/caregivers*.

800-MEDICARE (800-633-4227)
www.medicare.gov

National Institute on Aging Information Center (NIAIC)

Provides publications, information on clinical trials, links to other federal government agencies and organizations, and an online, searchable database of more than 300 organizations nationwide that provide help to older people.

P.O. Box 8250
Silver Spring, MD 20907
800-438-4380
301-495-3334 (TTY)
www.nia.nih.gov/alzheimers

NIHSeniorHealth *www.nihseniorhealth.gov*

Offers health and wellness information for older adults from the National Institute on Aging and the National Library of Medicine for older adults. Senior-friendly read-aloud and text features make it easy to use.

Legal and Financial Help

American Bar Association Commission on Law and Aging

Provides a state-by-state listing of resources available to help older persons with legal concerns and needs.

202-662-1000
www.abanet.org/aging/resources/statemap.shtml

BenefitsCheckUp.org *www.benefitscheckup.org*

Developed and maintained by the National Council on Aging (NCOA), BenefitsCheckUp.org helps find benefit programs for seniors with limited income and resources.

National Academy of Elder Law Attorneys

Provides information, education, and legal services to seniors and people with special needs.

1577 Spring Hill Road
Suite 220
Vienna, VA 22182
www.naela.org

Nolo *www.nolo.com*

Nolo Offers "plain-English" books, forms, and software, and affordable legal advice; tools to help you with wills, estate planning, retirement, eldercare, personal finance, taxes, housing and other legal concerns.

Reverse.org Consumer Information on Reverse Mortgages

www.reverse.org

Information on reverse mortgages.

UCompareHealthCare *www.ucomparehealthcare.com*

Free search for doctors, nursing homes, insurers; comparative data on health care institutions. A service of About.com.

Services

American Red Cross

Local chapters provide programs for older people, including safety courses and home nursing care instruction. Contact your local Red Cross office for senior care services.

2025 E Street NW
Washington, DC 20006
www.redcross.org

National Association of Professional Geriatric Care Managers

Search for a geriatric care manager by location.

3275 West Ina Road, Suite 130
Tucson, AZ 85741
520-881-8008
www.caremanager.org

Visiting Nurse Associations of America

Promotes home health education and helps search for home health services nationwide. Website offers suggested questions to ask service providers.

900 19th St. NW, Suite 200
Washington, DC 20006
202-384-1420
www.vnaa.org

Resources for Caregivers

ElderCare Online *www.ec-online.net*
Information, education and support for caregivers; safety advice; and links to additional caregiver resources.

Family Caregiver Alliance

National support, service, and advocacy organization publishes comprehensive information on legal, practical, and emotional aspects of caring for Alzheimer's; provides online caregiver instruction and tools and excellent, downloadable fact sheets on dementia, caregiving, and controlling frustration; hiring in-home help; and community care options.

180 Montgomery Street, Suite 1100
San Francisco, CA 94104
800-445-8106
www.caregiver.org

National Family Caregivers Association (NFCA)

Provides statistics, research reports, tip sheets, first-person accounts, a newsletter, and extensive resources and teleclasses.

10400 Connecticut Avenue, Suite 500
Kensington, MD 20895-3944
800-896-3650
www.nfcacares.org

FamilyCaregiving 101 *www.familycaregiving101.org*

NFCA's "how-to" site offers advice on time management, asking for help, navigating the health care maze, and more.

Well Spouse Association

Membership and advocacy organization focused on the needs of people caring for chronically ill and/or disabled spouses or partners.

63 West Main Street, Suite H
Freehold, NJ 07728
800-838-0879
www.wellspouse.org

Advocacy, Education, and Information

Alzheimer's Association
Offers a bounty of resources for individuals with AD, their families, and their caregivers. Operates a toll-free, 24/7 help line that provides reliable information, referrals, and support in several languages. Offers programs and services through local chapters; support groups; and online education and safety services. Sponsors MedicAlert + Alzheimer's Association Safe Return; Alzheimer's Association CareSource; and many other programs.

Alzheimer's Association National Office
225 N. Michigan Ave., Fl. 17
Chicago, IL 60601
800-272-3900
www.alz.org

Alzheimer's Foundation of America
National nonprofit organization providing information on Alzheimer's and other kinds of dementia, most of it geared toward caregivers rather than those with the disease. There are no local chapters; however, member organizations across the country provide services, such as consultation, education, identification bracelets, respite care, and support groups. You can search for your nearest member organization through the site.

Alzheimer's Foundation of America
322 8th Ave., 7th Fl.
New York, NY 10001
866-232-8484
www.alzfdn.org

National Hospice and Palliative Care Organization: Caring Connections

Nonprofit membership organization that provides state-specific information and advance directive documents for end-of-life care.

NHPCO
1731 King Street, Suite 100
Alexandria, VA 22314
703-837-1500
www.caringinfo.org

The National Citizens' Coalition for Nursing Home Reform (NCCNHR)

Provides guidance in selecting a quality nursing home and protecting residents' rights.

202-332-2275
www.nccnhr.org

Lewy Body Dementia Association

The second most common degenerative dementia after Alzheimer's disease, Lewy body dementia is little known, poorly understood, and frequently misdiagnosed. This organization offers the latest information about Lewy body dementia, support groups and forums, a newsletter, a help line and updates about clinical trials focusing on Lewy body dementia's causes and potential treatments.

912 Killian Hill Road SW, Suite 202C
Lilburn, GA 30047
National Office (Atlanta): 404-935-6444
Caregiver Helpline: 800-539-9767
www.lbda.org

Referral and Information Sources

AARP

AARP supplies information about caregiving, long-term care, and aging, including publications and audiovisual aids for caregivers.

601 E Street NW
Washington, DC 20049
888-687-2277
www.aarp.org

The AARP Guide to Internet Resources Related to Aging

This guide lists 300 sites and resources of interest to seniors. Print copies may be obtained by faxing a request to 202-434-6408 or writing to AARP, Research Information Center, 601 E Street NW, Washington, DC 20049. *www.aarp.org/internetresources*

HealthCentral Network *www.healthcentral.com*
Timely, in-depth medical information, personalized tools and resources, and connections to a vast community of leading experts and patients for people seeking to manage and improve their health.

Society for Neuroscience

Nonprofit membership organization of scientists and physicians who study the brain and nervous system.

1121 14th Street, Suite 1010
Washington, DC 20005
202-962-4000
www.ndgo.net/sfn/nerve

Centers for Disease Control and Prevention (CDC)

The federal government's center for research, development and application of disease prevention and control, environmental health, and health promotion and health education activities in the United States.

1600 Clifton Rd
Atlanta, GA 30333
404-639-3311
Public Inquiries: 404-639-3534 / 800-311-3435
www.cdc.gov/aging/info.htm

Mayo Clinic *www.mayoclinic.com*

A standard-bearer for quality medical care across the country, Mayo Clinic's encyclopedic website is arguably the most concise, accessible, and readable source of medical information on the web. Unlike many health sites, Mayo creates and produces its own material, which is written in an informative, sympathetic tone you will appreciate (particularly after slogging through the medical jargon and hype favored on so many sites).

Alzheimer Research Forum *www.alzforum.org*

Scientific, research, and treatment news and info.

Cochrane Collaboration *www.cochrane.org/reviews*

An international, independent, not-for-profit organization based in London that gathers, reviews, and publishes up-to-date, accurate information about the effects of health care worldwide. Reviewers are mostly health care professionals who volunteer to work in one of the many Cochrane Review Groups.

Fisher Center for Alzheimer's Research Foundation
www.alzinfo.org
Public-private collaboration for Alzheimer's research at New York's Rockefeller University.

MedlinePlus: Alzheimer's Disease
www.nlm.nih.gov/medlineplus/alzheimersdisease.html
Comprehensive online information from National Library of Medicine and National Institutes of Health.

Weblogs

Alzheimer's Reading Room
www.alzheimersreadingroom.com

Psychiatrist with Lewy Body Dementia
http://knittingdoc.wordpress.com

The Tangled Neuron: A Layperson Reports on Memory Loss, Alzheimer's & Dementia
www.tangledneuron.info

Recommended Books

Bell, Virginia, and David Troxel. *A Dignified Life: The Best Friends Approach to Alzheimer's Care: A Guide for Family Caregivers.* Deerfield Beach, FL: Health Communication, 2002.

Broyles, Frank. *Coach Broyles' Playbook for Alzheimer's Caregivers: A Practical Tips Guide.* Fayetteville, AR: University of Arkansas, 2006.

Coste, Joanne Koenig. *Learning to Speak Alzheimer's: A Groundbreaking Approach for Everyone Dealing with the Disease.* New York: St. Martin's Press, 2008.

Doraiswamy, P. Murali, and Lisa P. Gwyther. *The Alzheimer's Action Plan: The Experts' Guide to the Best Diagnosis and Treatment for Memory Problems.* With Tina Adler. New York: St. Martin's, 2008.

Halpern, Sue. *Can't Remember What I Forgot: The Good News from the Front Lines of Memory Research.* New York: Harmony Books, 2008.

Kuhn, Daniel and David Bennett. *Alzheimer's Early Stages: First Steps for Family, Friends, and Caregivers.* Alameda, CA: Hunter House, 2003.

Genova, Lisa. *Still Alice.* New York: Pocket Books, 2008. A neuroscientist's acclaimed first novel about a Harvard professor diagnosed with early-onset AD.

Mace, Nancy L., and Peter V. Rabins. *The 36-Hour Day: A Family Guide to Caring for Persons with Alzheimer's Disease, Related Dementing Illnesses, and Memory Loss in Later Life.* 3rd ed. Baltimore: Johns Hopkins University Press, 2006.

Peterson, Ronald. *Mayo Clinic on Alzheimer's Disease.* Rochester, MN: Mayo Clinic, 2004.

Ratey, John J. and Eric Hagerman *Spark: The Revolutionary New Science of Exercise and the Brain.* With Eric Hagerman. New York: Little, Brown, 2008.

Small, Gary. *The Memory Prescription: Dr. Gary Small's 14-Day Plan to Keep Your Brain and Body Young.* With Gigi Vorgan. New York: Hyperion, 2004.

Snowdon, David. *Aging with Grace: What the Nun Study Teaches Us about Leading Longer, Healthier, and More Meaningful Lives.* New York: Bantam, 2001.

Vaillant, George E. *Aging Well: Surprising Guideposts to a Happier Life from the Landmark Harvard Study of Adult Development.* Boston: Little, Brown, 2002.

Recommended Movies

Eyre, Richard, Charles Wood, and John Bayley. *Iris.* Directed by Richard Eyre. Starring Judi Dench, Jim Broadbent, Kate Winslet. West Hollywood, CA: Miramax Films, 2001.

Family Guide to Alzheimer's Disease. Five volumes. Directed by Mike Merryman. Hosted by Leeza Gibbons. Nashville, TN: LifeView Resources, Inc., 2004.

The Alzheimer's Project. Four-part documentary film series on AD first aired on HBO in May 2009. Films are part of a multi-platform public health series produced by the National Institute on Aging and HBO Documentary Films. Public health information and all films are available to view free at *www.hbo.com/alzheimers.*

Polley, Sarah. *Away from Her.* Adapted from *The Bear Came over the Mountain*, by Alice Munro. Directed by Sarah Polley. Starring Julie Christie, Gordon Pinsent. Canada: Mongrel Media, 2006.

Public Broadcasting System. *The Forgetting—A Portrait of Alzheimer's.* Documentary based on the book by David Shenk. Directed by Elizabeth Arledge. Narrated by David Hyde Pierce. St. Paul–Minneapolis: Twin Cities Public Television, 2004. Available online at *www.pbs.org/theforgetting.*

Index